For Pete & Ellen

Love —

Phyllis Adair

CLOSE, BUT NO CIGAR

A trip through the land of dementia

by

Phyllis O'Hara, ASN, BA, RNC (ret.)

Bloomington, IN Milton Keynes, UK

authorHOUSE®

AuthorHouse™
1663 Liberty Drive, Suite 200
Bloomington, IN 47403
www.authorhouse.com
Phone: 1-800-839-8640

AuthorHouse™ UK Ltd.
500 Avebury Boulevard
Central Milton Keynes, MK9 2BE
www.authorhouse.co.uk
Phone: 08001974150

First published by AuthorHouse 2/20/2007

ISBN: 978-1-4259-8582-0 (e)
ISBN: 978-1-4259-8581-3 (sc)

Printed in the United States of America
Bloomington, Indiana

This book is printed on acid-free paper.

Barkers… Carney workers at the turn of the century would tell those who tried to win at carnival games that they were "close" as they threw the ring or dart, but close didn't count. They would not receive the prize… often a cigar.

The goal of this book is to point out some of the situations often seen during that life span which includes diagnosis, denial, dreadful problems and death, as a result of dementia… usually in the form of Alzheimer's Disease.

Since hitting the mark… covering all of the various problems which caregivers and professionals alike face… is practically impossible, I know the cigar is out of reach. But honing skills gleaned from working with families and health professionals over the past twenty plus years, I'm going to try.

This is not intended to be either a scientific research source nor a "how to" advice book. If I have learned anything since I first started working in the field of Alzheimer's and other forms of dementia in 1983, it is that each case is different… each family has its own agenda… each physician, nurse, social worker, has their own body of knowledge and focus. "Cigar" is meant to be an adjunct to whatever classic publications you have already read. "The 36-Hour Day" is the seminal work of Peter Rabins and Nancy Mace. It has been the initial source of information for millions of caregivers. Their work has led to hundreds of fine volumes dealing with the physiologic changes in the brain of the dementia victim as well as many books which touch on the spiritual milieu of caregiving or on solving behavioral problems. Some are the personal stories of families who have coped with what dementia does to the whole family. Each volume adds to the body of work which has grown exponentially since Tomlinson, Blessed and Roth of the UK made their discovery in the late 1960s that Alzheimer's Disease was *not* restricted to those under age 55, as had been proposed by Alois Alzheimer in 1906.

I hope the information presented here will help to some degree those who come after me. If even one person gains enlightenment, knowledge, or a glimpse of a way to reach their loved one, then I truly will have 'the cigar'.

Phyllis O'Hara, ASN, BA, RN,C (ret.)
Greenfield, Massachusetts

To the families and caregivers
who taught me,

To the colleagues:
Carol, Kathy, Ginny, Sheila and Shirley

and the others:
The Bear, The Black Russian and The Jester
who supported me during difficult times.
And last, but always first, Ken

A Table of Contents
(more of less)

Where Do We Start? 1

The Mystery that is The Brain 5

So Who Is This Jon/Jan Q. Public?...........11

When Is It Dementia? 19

Who, Me? I Never Said That!....................27

"I've Got A Secret" 35

"The Steel Magnolia" That is the Mother................43

Olley, Olley, All's In Free! 49

"Slowly She Turned, Inch by Inch ..." 57

The Plot Thickens (Or is that 'a watched pot won't
    boil'?)..65

To Every Thing There is a Season? 77

"Old Timer's Disease" 81

Getting Back to "Old Timers" Disease 97

The Alphabet Soup People............................107

The Alphabet People 109

Another Tale or Two from this Storyteller's Bag....161

Continuing... and Then There Was Charlie...........167

There's GOT to be a Plan! 173

What Did I Forget? 185

Sources... Resources... On Line Sites 189

There are many people described in this book as having one disorder or another. Each individual is based in some part on people I have known or whose case was presented to me. All of the names, places, sexes, ages, families are part of my imagination. The only real person described is Uncle Charlie.

WHERE DO WE START?

This book has been arranged so that the reader will have an understanding of the beginnings of dementia and the signs and symptoms that might appear in the early stages. As an old professor once told me, "It's impossible to make decisions when you don't know what you are deciding!"

Pandora's box had nothing compared to the dementia box. Not only must we look at the physical brain and its workings, we also have to take a good hard look at some of the human behaviors which result because of things going on in the brain. I have no intention of trying to produce a treatise on the anatomy and physiology of the human brain. Neither training nor time would allow such an undertaking. But I can describe what we believe goes on in the brain of the patient with dementia and some of the current hypotheses: The 'How Comes' we need to know.

And so the first section of "Cigar" will be pretty much basic biology, a bit of chemistry and a lot of connecting the dots. Lydia Pinkham's Vegetable Compound has pretty much gone by the board, along with buggy

1

whips, eight-track tapes, disco and, I sincerely hope, "hardening of the arteries", getting "senile" and "gone loco."

It's 2006 as I write; families and other caregivers want to know many things about dementia while still referring to it as "confusion" or "some memory loss" or the ever popular "what do you expect? He's getting old!"

For a number of years in my 60s, I was a facilitator for the local Alzheimer's Disease Caregivers Support Group here in this rural western Massachusetts area. The members of the group taught me a great deal about what families go through in this seemingly unending role as caregiver for a dementia patient. To many, I gave a copy of "The Loss of Self" so that they might more easily understand their *own* role. As much as these meetings aided caregivers, it appeared that just telling people what they might expect didn't really cut the mustard when it came to real understanding. And so we will begin with a pretty cut and dried explanation of how the brain works, what happens when dementia enters the picture and how changes in the brain are expressed in the behaviors we see in the person.

There are many professionals who grimace when the word "patient" is used to describe the impaired person. I guess it's a kind of political incorrectness to use that term rather than 'loved one' or 'resident' or 'elder' person. Sorry, folks. They were patients to me for too many years, even when it was in my own family back in the 1930s.

So bear with me; this next chapter is about the nuts and bolts of the brain. It may be the final frontier that man will some day master. Right now, there is still mystery.

THE MYSTERY THAT IS THE BRAIN

How simple shall we make this?

The head is attached to the neck. I'm sure that comes as a big surprise. On the outside of the head there is skin with hair growing through the skin (in some people) and beneath that skin, the bony skull. Well, there is a membrane that keeps the brains from spilling out. Didn't you ever hear of a motorcycle helmet being described as a "brain bucket"? (Remember, I told you this was going to be very basic.)

The real "brains" are nerve cells (neurons) and a number of other cells that support the neurons. The actual neurons look like a starfish kind of thing with a central part called the cell body or nucleus. That's where your DNA and RNA live. The nerve cell or neuron has a bunch of branching arms that stick out from the main body. They're called dendrites. There is also a longer extension called the axon (it looks like a tail) that carries impulses from the cell body. This carrying is done by electricity.

So far, so good. Now, those dendrites, the branching arms or hairy things, receive messages from other dendrites. No, they don't have cell phones. But since the messages are carried by electricity, they can't just jump from one hairy dendrite to another. They need something in between; they need an infinitesimal chemical river!

Fascinating, isn't it! The chemicals found in the brain that do this work are called neurotransmitters... neuro meaning nerve and transmitters meaning just that. Sending. In this case, sending the electrical message from one hairy dendrite to the one next to it but not quite joined. Here comes the river part; the electric current which is carrying the message comes down the dendrite, reaches the neurotransmitter (chemical) river, and the message is picked up by the neurotransmitter and delivered to the hairy dendrite which is waiting to get the news... the electric thing.

Federal Express and Big Brown couldn't even *touch* this system!

But this is all done in microscopically infinitesimal size. Think of all the things of size that you know of. Like a mountain... or a whole city... or the State of Alaska (that being the largest of the 50, I believe)... and then think of a fingernail, or a mole. Now think of a germ. A bacterium is probably the largest germ we would see under a microscope.

Look at it this way. If I were a virus, then a building about 120 feet high would be a bacteria. It gets kind of overwhelming when you think of it that way. And if you were to look through a microscope at bacteria, you can see why you wouldn't see the virus through that same microscope. Too tiny. Electron microscopes are much better at this.

There are 10 billion to 100 billion neurons in the brain. There are 10 – 50 times that number of glial (supporting) cells. For a typical neuron, there are 1,000 to 10,000 synapses (those places where the message can be sent from one neuron to another).

All this material is jammed together in a folded, gelatin-like mass that fits inside the skull in sections which have been given names. Anterior means toward the front. The frontal lobe is located anterior to the rest of the brain. The temporal lobe is like the ear flaps of earmuffs. The parietal lobe is the connecting piece that holds the earmuff together. The occipital lobe is posterior, meaning to the back of the brain. These pieces put together form the cerebrum... the working part of the brain so that we can think, learn, remember, make decisions, and lots of other things.

Most of this working part is called the cerebral cortex and consists of the outer six layers of the cerebrum... that folded matter... and is often called the gray matter.

And the tail piece that connects with the spinal cord is known as the cerebellum. That's the part that controls your muscle coordination and balance among other things.

That's it for now. A good anatomy book from the library will cover all that I have left out. Let's go on to what happens when dementia enters the picture.

What? You don't want to know about dementia? That is probably because you really don't know about the medical words that are bandied about, hither and yon. About this time, some of you are wondering what kind of language is being used in this book! Remember, I'm an older adult, approaching seventy-seven years. That is a nice way of saying I'm pretty ancient to young people and I talk the way I learned back in the good old days.

We digress. Dementia is "a condition of declining mental abilities, especially memory. --- The person with dementia may also experience changes in personality, becoming aggressive, paranoid or depressed".

I can hear Aunt Bertha now telling me that what I described is just senility and to be expected in old people. You can tell that Aunt Bertha was *really* from the older generation.

Senescence: To age. Senile: To grow old. Senility: The process of aging. There is a difference. Part of the difference is cultural in that the word senile was given the additional meaning of losing one's mind or acting in a senile manner. Tell people long enough that senile means dementia and they will start to believe it.

It is true that as we age there are changes in our body and mind. Aging is partly responsible for increased numbers of cataracts in the eye (clouding of the lens) and a decrease in the ability to hear certain sounds or tones of voices. Most people have a loss of some hair, drying and thinning of the skin, muscle decrease (except for those gym rats that have learned that you *don't* have to lose it!). There is also a loss in lung capacity, decreases in the gastrointestinal tract (that's why you have to watch your medications) and a slowing of function in both liver and kidneys. Oops. Technical!

Why is it that some people reach age 55 or 60 and believe that life, for them, is over and they might just as well give up on everything? And at the same time, we find people who take on entirely new lives or occupations, sometimes becoming more proficient in their second life/occupation than in their first?

The human "homo sapiens"... our title in the evolutionary table... is a marvelous creature making use of the various mental and physical capabilities which are part and parcel of being a human. So how come it seems that so many of these people are willing to put it all away when a few symptoms of aging set in?

Before we get to the nitty-gritty of what dementia does to the brain, I'd like to tell you a few things about how this body copes with aging. Sort of the "Rise and Fall of Jon/Jan Q. Public."

So Who Is This Jon/Jan Q. Public?

The mythical man in the street used to be quoted by radio newscasters with the words "according to John Q. Public ..." I often wondered if they really did go into the streets to poll the people.

But since Jon/Jan, for political correctness, are the general public in this millennia, I'll treat them as the normal older adult for our purposes.

If you are speaking of the older adult at this time in the history of man, you would have to be pretty specific as to which decade of life you are referring. Many years ago, say around the turn of the 20th century, the average life span of a man in the United States would have been about 49 years. Obviously we have come a long way since then. Adults today live into their late 70s and a very large majority into the frame of the "oldest old" which encompasses those 85+. This situation turns out to be a major contributor to the exponential rise in the Alzheimer's Disease diagnosis. "How come?" as my old friend Ben used to say.

Ben was a car dealer and he often remarked that after selling a car, the owner would invariably be back to see him with the question, "How come ...?" In his case, the 'how comes' usually referred to questions already answered and, in fact, were readily available in the book which came with the car.

When Alois Alzheimer first gave his name to the form of dementia he saw in a woman seen by him for treatment, he described all the classic signs of dementia. However, this woman was 55 years old. Perhaps we can safely say that in 1906 when this event occurred, the woman was old.

When Tomlinson, Blessed and Roth published their "Observations on the brains of non-demented old people" in 1968, the whole picture changed. This group from the United Kingdom had published work previously pointing out that it appeared that Alzheimer's was *not* just a 'pre-senile' dementia (coming before the older ages) but was indeed the same disorder which Alzheimer himself had described in 1906. (In later years, Barry Reisberg, M.D., himself a giant in the field of Alzheimer research, would comment that the 1968 report in the Journal of Science was 'a classic article which would become an important historical document.')

What does this all mean in simple language? That Alzheimer's Disease (AD) is a brain disorder which usually is found in older adults but can be found in younger people as well. It also means that the reason we didn't hear very much about AD until the last twenty-five years (this being the 25th anniversary of the Alzheimer's Association) was first... people weren't living long enough for the disease to 'kick in' and died of other ailments before that time, and second... the disease itself wasn't fully described as to age of onset until the boys from across the pond told the world about their discovery.

That's all well and good, you say. But how come aging has something to do with AD? That's a horse of another color. (So now she's playing games with Shakespeare?)

Let's look at it this way: There are many changes associated with aging. Among the noticeable are... loss of height. Most all older adults are shorter than in their twenties. The combination of those vertebrae and discs compressing causes the loss of height and often the stooped posture among those with osteoporosis.

Then we often have decreased weight because of metabolism and decreased total water in the cells. Some might point out that we are in an epidemic of obesity as I write... but watch those people in their 90s and see if the 'norm' isn't true.

Skin problems galore: wrinkles, thinning skin and dryness which accounts for so many skin 'tears' in some elders. Things like 'skin tags' and 'senile keratoses' along with cherry hemangiomas. WHAT? Ask your physician. None of them are going to cause you much trouble so we choose to ignore them.

The heart and the rest of the cardiovascular system... arteries, veins, etc., have some changes that are serious and some that we can just live with. Many elders are on medications for high blood pressure, high cholesterol, changes in heart beat, and other such drugs. We've come to expect it in older adults, although there are a number of very healthy people who approach their 80s and even the 90s with few pills on their plate. But it is true that the heart can't put out the blood to the organs as easily as in youth. The heart rate itself may decrease. There may be thickening in the arteries from plaque, so well described on any television commercial. (Maybe there *is* some good from all those pill ads.)

Kidney function includes the rest of the tubing, etc. that makes the urinary tract work. Men, in particular are going to be faced with enlargement of the prostate gland (that is *not* 'prostrate' which means lying full length, face down) just so you won't be confused about this. The gland gets bigger with age and obstructs the flow of urine in men. Prostate cancer, too, increases dramatically with age. It's a good thing men are now having the 'digital exam' and the blood test for their 'prostate specific antigen' which allows your physician/ health provider to keep an eye on the status of that situation. And don't think women get off easy. There is an increase in urinary tract infections in older women. We can't win!

The human liver has many roles to play; we are looking at the ability of the liver to continue its normal work while being overloaded with medications which need to be cleared by either the kidneys or liver or both. Here's the story. As we age, the blood flow to the liver decreases. In turn, this has a large affect on how drugs (some more than others) are cleared from the system. The decrease may be in the range of 30 – 40%, Many drugs have what is called "active metabolites" which may remain in the body in a concentrated form. Some can actually cause toxicity.

Now you add to that decreased liver function a change in renal (kidney) blood flow too and you can see that certain drugs may be hanging around in the system of the older adult. That is one reason why doctors who start a patient on a new drug will say, "Start low and go slow."

What else can go wrong in the body of Jon and Jan?

I'm sure we are all aware of changes in hearing acuity with age. Some women believe that their husbands have selective hearing loss, primarily when it is their wife who is doing the speaking and the husband *never heard her say such a thing.* Seriously, there are many changes in our hearing apparatus which may be causing the inability to hear certain tones or to discriminate between sounds. I can attest to this difficulty. My own hearing is extremely good. I once asked my husband to look outside on a summer evening to see if it had started to rain. He returned to tell me that a neighbor three houses down had their sprinkler on. On the other hand, heeding the reminder to check the smoke alarms when daylight savings starts and ends had a startling response from same husband. I was testing the button and couldn't stop the alarm from screeching. I asked him to please take the alarm down so I could take the battery out to stop the horrible noise. "What noise?" Unbelievable! I had him come into the front hall and I plugged the alarm back in. I couldn't stand it... but he didn't hear it!

Fortunately, our local Fire Department has a program for people like Ken, who, even with bilateral hearing aids, cannot hear a smoke alarm. We now have a special alarm in our bedroom which has one of those blinding white lights that announce the detection of smoke. It also has an alarm to wake the dead, as my dear old mother used to say. Must be an Irish phrase; I know it appears in a play by James Joyce.

So now we know that hearing may or may not be affected by age. We also know, or certainly are aware in some manner, that there are changes in our eyes. It may be that 'your arms aren't long enough to read the phone book' as a friend in his early 50s once said. Reading glasses become necessary for some. Or bifocals for those who have needed distance glasses for many years. Then there is the lack of color sharpness, of lines of demarcation, and problems with depth perception. We know about cataracts and, I certainly hope, that all know of the new surgeries to correct this condition, bringing remarkable results. I couldn't believe how sharp the colors in nature were after having lens replacements in both eyes. I was also delighted to know that I no longer need glasses to drive and can, with patience, read without glasses. My drug store specials (magnifiers) do the job when I start serious reading. Macular degeneration, glaucoma and retinal detachment are serious eye problems which need immediate attention. Part of aging, I suppose. These two are serious problems which can lead to blindness. In a later chapter I'll talk about the changes in vision which occur with Alzheimer's. This is a subject which has been the topic of a great deal of research in more recent years.

I'm not through yet. Taste buds decrease. Osteoarthritis becomes more prominent. Lungs don't have the power they had in our teen years. There is a lack of elasticity in the lungs (normal with aging to some extent) and more and more we face COPD … chronic obstructive pulmonary disease. Perhaps with the realization in younger folks that smoking can really mess up your life in later years, COPD will not be the direct result of tobacco. There are, of course, other causes of COPD, but the bronchial asthma, emphysema and other nasties are, for the most part, the present left for us by the tobacco companies.

Thus, Jon and Jan have many things to face as they age. We have recently learned that weight training can be very helpful in even the old-old. Walking is now the activity 'de jour' for all; there are walking groups and 'mall walkers' have become a part of the social scene. Winter weather won't keep these folks from their appointed date with the 'mall-before-opening' across the country.

The one thing we haven't touched on is the aging brain.

How does the brain change as we age? Isn't it normal to have loss of memory in old age? Isn't this loss, and the more serious losses of dementia to be expected if you live long enough?

I wish Marion was still alive. One early winter day as I drove by her house, I stopped to admonish her for her activity: she was shoveling snow. She was also approaching 100. Do you know how many centenarians there are in the U.S.? One source reports there were 37,000; another source points out that since birth certificates were not universal until the 1930s, we may be looking at a number of people 110 or older.

Being well and active at 100 is wonderful. But being 100 and having no idea who you are or even being able to communicate is not wonderful. And we will talk about that next.

WHEN IS IT DEMENTIA?

Now that we know physical conditions can cause memory problems aside from those of true dementia, I'd like to talk about the young guy who gets our memories from the back of the storeroom. I've spoken about him at various presentations over the past twenty years so I'm sure some of you have heard his story.

When we are younger, say under thirty, we never seem to have a problem recalling a fact or a face. I understand that certain young people, however, seem quite able to remember every line of a rap but find homework and class work impossible to recall. At least that was the situation with my five offspring.

Something seems to happen as we age and it really has nothing to do with dementia. It's called the slowdown in our retrieval system. This is where my imaginary young guy comes in. You see, when we were young, he was in perfect physical shape, made even better by his newest shoes. I'm not sure which company he favored, but Nike and Air Jordan or something comes to mind. You wanted to remember something and, like a flash, it was right there at the tip of your tongue or in front of your eyes. Magical!

Age takes a toll on this young guy. We hit fifty... he hits fifty. We aren't as quick as we used to be... neither is he! What slows him down getting to those memory banks so that he can get that important stuff to us? Slow down in the retrieval system! Remember; electricity... chemicals... brain cells? Those chemicals have a tendency to decrease somewhat with age and unless we have the system working at full speed, we have to wait for the answer to get processed so that 'we remember'!

Haven't you had this kind of an experience: you are in the super market, following your list, pushing that cart through the aisles and this woman comes toward you, a smile on her face, as she says, "It's so good to see you! I hope things are going better for you now."? Panic time. You can't for the life of you remember her name, although her face is very familiar. Who is she? How do you know her? (All this time, thinking you must have developed Alzheimer's.)

So you politely make the shortest version of small talk... trying to say a few words that would allow you to get on your way without appearing to be a total dolt.

"Oh, yes. It's good to see you, too. I'm in quite a rush today... have an appointment I must get to. We'll talk later." As you hurry up the aisle. Familiar?

You are about to check out when, the "AH HA" strikes. Ah, ha; she was a neighbor of your sister-in-law and you last saw her at your niece's baby shower. Her name is ...

This is not the same as walking into your kitchen and staring at the refrigerator, then the cupboards, saying "What did I come in here for?"

That one happens to young and old. Perhaps a bit of broken concentration? Thinking about more important things and the thought that brought you to the kitchen kind of drifted off into space?

Or maybe you are a crossword puzzle aficionado who can't wait to get to that daily puzzle with your coffee. You've been doing the puzzle in this paper for so long that you can snap right through it. But the paper seems to be using another puzzle maker and the puzzle is a bit harder. It may be just a bit different rather than harder. You go to it and ... "what the heck is that word ... used to be a player in that TV show ... did a few movies" ... AH HA, again. It may be that it took you to the end of the puzzle to get it, but you were successful.

Retrieval system at work again. But in some cases, there is no AH HA.

In some older adults, the AH HA never comes. There is a fine line between the small loss of memory which is normal for people over 75 (some say over 70) and that which has been designated as "mild cognitive impairment" in the recent literature.

Mild cognitive impairment (MCI... and not the phone company) may very well be the early-early start of Alzheimer's. Research studies in the past five years indicate that when individuals have been diagnosed with MCI, they more often than not go on to full blown Alzheimer's. But where is the line here?

Alzheimer's disease is not just memory loss. There are a number of things which may be out of kilter in the brain of the AD patient. Not only do they have a problem with recent memory, dementia patients exhibit poor judgment; they have problems with abstract thinking and often show a lack of initiative.

Later, I'll refer to the Alzheimer's Association list of the "Ten Warning Signs" of AD. But now we're looking at either memory deficits normal for a person say, 83 years old or apparent MCI. Here's my problem with these two descriptions.

Your normal 83 year old man (same for women but we'll start with the guy) can be an active, youthful tennis player who prides himself on his low cholesterol, lack of cardiac problems and general upbeat personality. He admits he sometimes has a problem remembering the name of someone whom he has only seen in business meetings. He does have a PDA on which he depends to structure most of his life and believes we should take advantage of modern methods. His wife reports that she thinks he is slowing down because he sometimes can't find the right word when he is speaking with her. She admits, however, that he can usually express himself by using another word, or can wait to have the word come to mind. Normal? Or is this MCI?

Another 83 year old man was never active in sports although he does walk every day and remarks that his father's "constitutional" probably had some bearing on his choice of activity. He has been a Type II diabetic for about fifteen years and monitors his blood level faithfully four times a day. Knowing that heart, kidney and eye problems can be affected by diabetes, he watches his diet, eats according to his dietary plan and makes certain that he sees his ophthalmologist every year. He retired at age 65 and has spent most of his retirement years traveling with his wife to visit children and grand kids. At 83, he has decided to let his wife do most of the driving. He found that he sometimes didn't recognize the right turnoff on the interstate and gets upset when he is challenged by changes in the usual route. He is a bit less sociable since he turned 80 but still gets to church every Sunday and enjoys his Men's Group. He admits that he is slowing down, but "doesn't everyone at my age?" Another MCI? Or just normal?

The first man is an example of someone who is fortunate to have such good health. He obviously has worked to keep himself in good shape. Keeping cholesterol and triglycerides in check has been noted as a possible way of staving off AD. His wife's description of 'slowing down' appears to be more of a statement of her own concerns, in that even this mild event, in her mind, may look like early stage dementia.

As for our second man, he may have more trouble down the road. Diabetes mellitus is a serious physical disorder which can lead to problems in the brain as well as in the heart, kidneys and eyes. There have been several studies noting that so called brittle diabetes in itself can account for a degree of dementia. Recognizing that he has concerns about his driving shows that his judgment is probably still good. The lack of sociability might be taken as a loss of initiative, another possible sign of dementia. In this case, we might find that his withdrawal from previously enjoyed activities may be either a sign of oncoming dementia or a sign of depression, not previously diagnosed.

This would be a good stopping point. Let's look at the Alzheimer's Association's list of "The Ten Warning Signs of Alzheimer's Disease."

1] Memory loss
2] Difficulty performing familiar tasks
3] Problems with language
4] Disorientation to time and place
5] Poor or decreased judgment
6] Problems with abstract thinking
7] Misplacing things
8] Changes in mood or behavior
9] Changes in personality
10] Loss of initiative

While many elders have some of these warning signs, it is also necessary to determine whether the signs are truly indicative of early stage dementia or are side effects of some other biological problem in the person.

This is a personal note. I wonder if, when putting a diagnostic label on a small memory problem, should that incidence be then folded into the MCI diagnosis? Does the fact that there is memory involved without other supporting diagnostic deficits help the person with the loss, or does it help the person doing the diagnosing?

Can naming "early dementia" cause a cascade of anxiety, fear, guilt and hopelessness in the patient? Can these symptoms push an already fragile person into depression? Is it wiser to keep our thoughts on the matter to ourselves while scheduling more frequent appointments with the individual?

Dementia, mild cognitive impairment or a bit of slippage in the older adult; there is much to be discovered about delineating lines when it comes to diagnosis.

WHO, ME?
I NEVER SAID THAT!

Y ou are going to meet a large number of people
in this book. Well populated book: every one
has a first name and a last initial (I'm being much
more careful) and don't be surprised it the first name
is followed by a last name with the alphabetical letter
which would follow the first initial of the first name.
Are you totally confused? Then I will tell you about
Alice B and her friend Carla D. Got it?

Alice B is a school teacher. Her friend, Carla D,
teaches at the same school and the two women have
been close friends for forty years. Both widowed, they
often spend their recreational time, holidays, vacation
weeks and summer vacations, together. Since neither
woman has close family, the situation has allowed them
to have a dependable person in their lives while still
being able to maintain their private home life.

Forty years is a long time to be a teacher, particularly
in this day and age. Retirement is on the agenda for
both women, probably in two years. Carla, however,
has become increasingly concerned about Alice and

certain changes she has seen in her over the past year or so. Carla knows that Alice has one daughter who lives some two hundred miles from the small town in which both women teach. But does she have the right to contact the daughter (Eliza F) to voice her concerns?

Here is the situation: While driving to the Cape in August, just prior to the opening day of school, Alice made a wrong turn and ended up heading for Boston instead of Cape Cod. When Carla commented on the mistake, Alice became extremely angry and accused Carla of telling her to take the route on which they found themselves. Rather than cause a commotion, Carla went along with Alice, hoping that she would see her mistake when she came across a familiar landmark.

So, instead of heading southeast to the Cape, they were on a northeasterly highway. When the signs for Plymouth Rock came into view, Alice started to berate Carla, accusing her of trying to confuse her and of having the ulterior motive of not wanting to go to the Cape in the first place.

Are you totally confused? Carla was. To make matters worse, Alice refused to turn back. She said that Carla had told her yesterday that she really didn't want to go to the Cape for the weekend. To which Carla, of course, replied, "Who me? I never said that!"

If this had been the only incident which had caused Carla to have an uneasy feeling, she wouldn't have even considered informing Eliza. There was also the incident over the Fourth of July when Alice had invited all the teachers in their elementary school to come to her home for a cookout and to watch the fireworks from her front porch. Carla had offered to come to the house in the middle of the afternoon to help Alice prepare for the supper.

Arriving at Alice's home at about 4:00 p.m., she discovered that Alice was nowhere to be found. Her car was gone and, from all appearances, she hadn't started any preparations for the evening event. Peering into the kitchen window, she noted that the room was disorganized and that there were no bags, cartons, boxes or other hints that there was to be a supper here.

The guests were to arrive at 6:00 p.m. When Alice had not returned by 5:30, Carla decided to leave a note on the door asking that all teachers convene at her home, about two streets distant. She then headed out for the super market to gather supplies for an impromptu meal.

Carla was busily setting the picnic table on her patio when the first guests arrived. Since there would only be about ten people, it wasn't hard to put together a substitute celebration. Everyone took a chore and by 7:00, all were eating and drinking, without a clue as to what had happened to their missing colleague.

The fireworks started at 9:00 and the oooooooos and aaaaaaahhhhs went on until the grand finale. At least they thought it was the grand finale. Not to be. Alice arrived. Oh, boy; did she ever arrive!

Looking back at that event, Carla said, "I probably should have recognized that she was in a state of pure paranoia! First she accused me of getting all our friends to come to my house without inviting her. She went on and on about how none of us appreciate her and that she couldn't understand why we all hated her."

By the time the other teachers tried to talk with Alice, it became pretty apparent that there was nothing (and no one) which could pacify her. It also became clear that she had absolutely no memory of having invited all to her house for the celebration.

That ended the fireworks of the 4th for the teachers group. Everyone left in an embarrassed state, not knowing what to say or how to handle the situation. Can you imagine this group of ten well educated, emotionally stable adults being totally unable to help Carla as she tried to placate Alice?

So we have two rather obvious incidents in which Alice was just not Alice. There were other episodes of memory loss, including one in which she neglected to get her report cards in to the Principal's office on time. She was spoken to rather sharply by the boss lady who tried to get to the bottom of the problem. Not realizing what the rest of the staff knew, she only succeeded in making Alice more angry, defensive and petulant.

When the fall semester started, Carla went to the Principal and told her about the two events which had occurred over the summer. This whole thing got tangled up in the 'rights and responsibilities' of the school in such a matter. Do we tell? Who do we tell? Can we be sued for making false claims? Now here's a fine kettle of fish!

I won't bother you with all the details which included speaking to the attorney for the school department and several other steps. Finally cleared for take off... Carla called Eliza.

Change of scenery: Eliza F has come to a small restaurant outside of the town where her mother lives.

She was to meet with Carla to talk about the situation with mother Alice.

Eliza was a thirty-five year old married mother of two who still worked part time as a nurse in a hospital in central New York State. Because of her multiple family obligations, she was not a frequent visitor in her mother's home. Her family would pack up the kiddoes and the holiday gifts the Sunday before Christmas and drive to Grandmas... sort of like the 'over the river and through the woods' written by another Massachusetts women.

Last holiday visit, Eliza had noticed that the house was in disarray, something totally out of character for her mother. Alice simply explained that she had been doing extra projects at the school and that had taken up her time. Alice had become quite adept at making up stories to cover whatever came up. The grandchildren had been told to be very quiet at the house because Grandma didn't like noise. This, too, was out of character for Alice who had always looked forward to having the children come for a visit.

Eliza told Carla that her mother had been calling her nearly every day asking why she didn't come to see her. This certainly didn't make any sense knowing the distance between the two homes. But Eliza had just put it off to the back of her mind, thinking that whatever was the problem, another day or two wasn't going to make any difference.

That meeting at the restaurant lasted nearly three hours. Good thing the proprietors were friends of the school staff!

Carla reported on the two main incidents: July 4th and the Cape Cod non-trip. She then asked Eliza if she knew anything about her mother's physical situation... any illness that she knew of that might cause these problems. Eliza, however, didn't even know if her mother had a doctor! Or is that 'personal care provider' in 2006 terms?

What came out of the meeting might remind some of you of what is known as "Intervention" in the field of alcoholism. All the family and friends get together and confront the afflicted person, the goal being to discover what is going wrong and how those nearest and dearest can point out solutions or routes to follow.

Carla, the Principal of the school, Eliza and a minister with whom Alice was comfortable all showed up at Alice's home, unannounced. In retrospect, the family now believes that this method was probably too strident for a woman who was treading water as fast as she could in order to stay afloat. But at that time, the BIG "A" WORD hadn't been voiced.

As might have been expected, the paranoia which had been noticed on previous occasions came to the forefront of the conversation. Alice denied any problems with her memory, even when specific incidents were mentioned. She denied having invited people to the 4th party. She denied having told Carla that she had taken the wrong turn. She denied ever having been late passing in report cards. She practically denied having a daughter!

The extraneous people were given leave and Eliza, Carla and Alice sat down to talk about medical problems which might or might not exist. Eliza was stunned to learn that her mother had not seen a physician for nearly twenty years. And all this time, she thought her mother was getting annual physicals, having mammograms, checking her cholesterol and other important components of a good physical. (That's probably why they say that to assume is to make an ass of 'u' and me.)

Alice was very cool to Carla, realizing that she was probably the source of all this which was being put upon her. She didn't think too kindly of Eliza, either! But she did agree to have Eliza make an appointment with a physician... her previous M.D. having been deceased for some ten years.

Eliza had made arrangements to stay with her mother for the remainder of the week. She then started looking into mother's legal and financial affairs, hoping that perhaps whatever was causing the memory problems didn't spill over into the other aspects of her life. The spillage was more like a flood.

How could this woman have continued teaching while the rest of her life was a total morass of difficulties? There were bills unpaid, including the real estate tax on the house. There was a notice of cancellation of services on both her electric and telephone service. It appeared that she had not paid her oil bill for last winter... at least not the last half of it. As she discovered more and more segments of her mother's life that were in a state of limbo, Eliza realized that just seeing a doctor wasn't going to do much to solve the multiple problems that were becoming quite obvious.

So as we close this chapter of "Alice Faces Life" or "Eliza Becomes the Mother" we turn to the medical visit and what happened… should have happened… and didn't happen!

"I've Got A Secret"

Let's see... Garry Moore, Bill Cullen, Steve Allen, and there was Arlene Francis, Henry Morgan, Dorothy Kilgallen, Kity Carlisle and a host of others. Does this all seem unfamiliar? Then you weren't around during the "Golden Age of Television" when Goodson and Todman ruled the airwaves with their various shows.

The idea of the show was to have three persons come on stage and announce to the blindfolded panel members, "My name is Joe Doaks,' also repeated by the other two persons. The panelists would then ask questions and try to guess which person was actually the 'celebrity' guest. If the true "Joe Doaks" had an easily recognizable name, that would entail a voice change or an accent added, just to confuse the panelists. Actually, it was great fun, long before the reality style television of the more recent years.

These were definitely not demented individuals but their ability to act out the role of another person added to the fun of the show. This, however, is not the case when an individual comes to the office of their physician or other healthcare provider, in many cases, with some reticence.

These men and women approach the idea of having a physical examination (which will probably also include some degree of cognitive testing) with about as much glee as the six year old having dental work done. Fighting and dragging may not fully describe the true situation. But if you can picture a thirty-something daughter or a forty-plus son trying to get the parent to accept the fact that a complete physical is an absolute necessity, with a negative response from the older adult, you may appreciate the problem.

This is where we find that "I've Got A Secret" had nothing on mother or father when it comes to answering the probing questions of the doctor. The offspring who have seen the decline in the parent are not prepared to find that said parent has suddenly become another person!

Alice wasn't really too keen on going to a doctor after the twenty year hiatus. And of course she didn't like it that Eliza had chosen a woman physician. Doctors are men and women are nurses. The invisible chip on Alice's shoulder told all present that this was not going to be a pleasant occasion.

But since she was there, Alice decided to fake everybody out. She was able to schmooze her way through questions by turning the question back on the person who first queried. "Now, Mrs. B., how have you been feeling?"

"Perfectly fine and dandy!" replied Alice. "I watch my weight and walk every day. I know what they say on television about keeping active. I don't take any pills and don't need any."

Dr. G then told her that she would do a complete physical, have some blood drawn so that they could learn if there was any deviation from normal, do an ECG to check her heart, and then take it from there.

Alice was as sweet as could be. She agreed completely and then told the doctor that she was actually the one who wanted to come to the office. "My daughter thought I should see someone, but I was really the one who brought up the subject," Alice continued.

Eliza's jaw had been at half mast since her mother started to talk but decided that putting in her two cents wasn't going to help. She did, however, tell the doctor that she and some of Alice's friends had some concerns about her memory and certain events which had taken place during the preceding six months or more.

"Mother was to host a fourth of July event this year but evidently forgot all about the fact that she had asked her friends to come to her house."

Alice jumped right in, saying, "It wasn't that I forgot anything. There were no such plans ever made," she said. "Furthermore, I can't understand why my friends would think that I would have such a gathering, knowing that I hadn't planned to be at home that day."

(I must interject here: I can't tell you how many times I have been told by family members that, while standing or sitting out of the parents sight, they have had to mouth the words "No, No, No" while waving their arms over their head as the parent invented stories with absolutely no factual content.)

Alice continued. The smile on her face belied the anger she was attempting to hold back. "And while I'm here, I do think you should know that my friend Carla has been telling some of the teachers that my work at school isn't up to par. That's a flat out lie and I can't imagine why she continues to say such things."

The wise Dr. G changed the subject. "Now Alice … may I call you Alice?" She received a nod of approval from the ever-smiling subject.

"I'd like to ask you a few questions. Nothing hard, you understand. "

"Where did you go to school?" she asked.

Alice responded: "I attended a school up in the hills. It was a small school and not many children belonged to that particular school."

Eliza nodded in agreement from her somewhat hidden spot.

"And where did you go after that school? asked Dr. G.

"After that school… let me see … I must have been about seventeen then. My parents wanted me to go to work so I moved closer into the town and went to work in a factory."

Here came the waving arms, the mouthed "No" and the waving arms accompanied by the head shaking, indicating that we had hit a major error in the life history.

Dr. G., ever aware of the ins and outs of confabulation (a spontaneous production of false information which may or may not be caused by failing memory or the need to fill in the blanks where a memory should have been).

"And do you have children, Alice?'

Yes. My daughter, Eliza. But she doesn't live around here. I'm not sure where she does live. I think she got married." Turning to Eliza, she asked, "Didn't you get married or something?"

"Yes, Mother," Eliza replied, "I was married and..." the doctor interrupted, indicating that she wanted no further input from the daughter.

Addressing Alice again, "Do you work?"

Back in control, discussing a familiar subject, Alice replied, "I've been a teacher for quite a number of years now. I plan to retire in a year or so. I'm pretty tired of teaching the same children and same subjects, year after year."

Once again, an interruption. The fact that Alice could continue to teach without really "blowing it" was probably because of the routine which continued day in and day out, year after year. She taught very young children and the curriculum and class plan continued like a broken record, monotonously flowing throughout her life. Had Alice suddenly been asked to fill in for another teacher during the preceding two years or so, the staff would have been very aware of her shortcomings much sooner. Structure, though dull, played in her favor.

Returning to the questioning, Dr. G said, "I'm going to give you three words and I would like you to repeat them to me. Blue, paper, kitten."

"Blue, kitten, paper," said Alice. Still smiling. Still in control, so she thought.

Dr .G again. "Now, Alice, I know you're a teacher so this one is easy. Spell WORLD backward."

It came out "D O R W"... still smiling.

"Fine. Now I would like you to count from 100 backward, by 7s."

Alice was able to get to 93, but the next number was 90, then 85. A bit of a problem here, wouldn't you say?

Dr. G then talked to Alice about what she had for breakfast that morning. This is the easiest question for many elders who have the same identical meal every day. While it may be a logical question, the answers don't usually amount to a hill of beans. But Alice thought this would be a great way to really snow the doctor.

"I love my coffee. And while orange juice is a good morning drink, I usually have grape juice, or if I'm making pancakes, I won't have any juice. Then I make sure I have an egg. I think that a well balanced meal is important, don't you? Bacon isn't good for your heart so I have fried fish. Then I cook a few vegetables, depending on what hits my fancy."

That didn't even get a response from Eliza, who sat shaking her head in disbelief.

"Now, Alice… I told you three words earlier. Can you tell me what they were?"

"Of course, I can. You told me bacon, school and summer." The smile this time was on the face of Dr. G.

"Well, well, now. You certainly have been answering all my questions. There is one other thing I'd like you to do. I would like you to draw the face of a clock, write the correct numbers on the face, and then show the time with two arrows at 10:25."

Those of you who do not know about the clock face drawing test may not realize that this one test can tell you a great deal more about your patient than all the other tests combined. At least that has been the report of many who work in the field of dementia. In the case of our friend Alice, the results were pretty much what Dr. G expected.

Alice drew what looked a bit like an egg standing on its broad base. The '1' was at the top of the egg, and the numbers through 9 were written down the right hand side of the clock. The 10 was at the base and there were a jumble of numbers going up the left side. Those included 13, 14, 15. The arms or number indicators were one broad black arrow aimed at the bottom of her clock… meaning, I guess, that was the 'ten' needed for the test.

Dr. G thanked Alice for her help and patience and told her that the paper work to have her laboratory tests would be given to Eliza to take home. As Alice walked out of the office, Dr. G nodded to Eliza and said, "I'll send you a detailed report and suggestions. You, of course, already know the answer."

The enlightening afternoon was over and while Alice was convinced that she had done a remarkable job (indeed she had!) it was Eliza who was faced with the realization that she had an enormous job ahead.

How on earth could this woman be so completely confused and yet appear to be perfectly normal? Yes, there were the unpaid bills… that would be up to Eliza to straighten out… and there would undoubtedly be other legal and financial matters to discuss… but how could she possibly manage to convince her mother that she would have to give up teaching immediately and probably wouldn't be able to drive her car. How could she handle her own family, so far away yet so near, and still keep her mother safe?

Why couldn't she have had a sibling with whom she could share the burden! Welcome to the world of Alzheimer's... the world in which everything can appear to be fine yet there is an empty space behind that pleasant façade.

"THE STEEL MAGNOLIA" THAT IS THE MOTHER

That movie was always one of Alice's favorites. Alice had a steel will, I know that. She didn't bend... on any subject.

While it is probably true that many of us get 'set in our ways' as the years pass, there is a certain stubbornness seen in older adults when dementia enters the picture. I do not attribute this trait only to women. I have seen men whose inability to condescend to the wishes of those who care for them has been just as strong, if not stronger, than some women.

Alonzo K. was one such man. But Alice, I believe, had him beat, hands down. (The tale of Al and Mac comes later.)

When Eliza returned to her mother's home, she was well aware that she had a huge job ahead and that she would be the one to take on this chore. Her plan was to talk with Alice, get an idea of what legal and financial matters needed attention and then start making the necessary contacts. But first, she put a call through to her husband to let him know that she wouldn't be coming home for at least the remainder of the week. Fortunately, the hospital where she worked wasn't short staffed at the time and they understood her predicament.

Rather than jump into what might be a sticky morass, she asked Alice if she would like to go out for dinner at her favorite restaurant. She thought this might be a way to calm the waters, so to speak. Alice was no longer smiling. In fact, she was pretty icy!

"Well, I hope you're satisfied," she said. "All your talk about there being something wrong with me and that doctor woman didn't find anything wrong!"

Eliza was flabbergasted, to say the least. She was totally surprised at her mother's belief that there was nothing wrong with her. How could she believe that? Couldn't she see that there had been numerous mistakes made in the testing?

Sometimes it is hard for adults to tell other adults the truth. Dr. G had been extremely careful in her conversations during the testing procedure. But she had quickly glossed over any of Alice's mistakes, going on to the next part of the test as though Alice had been correct in each of her answers. It might have been better if she had carefully couched her words, giving Alice at least some indication that she was experiencing problems with her brain function. Eliza wasn't the person to tell her mother that she had not done well on the mental status exam. But since Dr. G had failed to even mention the errors, it appeared that Eliza had more of a job than anticipated.

Alice flounced off into the kitchen, banging pots and pans, running the water, slamming the cupboard doors and having an adult level tantrum. When Eliza followed her mother to the kitchen, Alice screamed at her, "Get out of my house. You aren't my daughter. You are trying to take my life away from me!"

"That's another fine mess you've gotten us into," was a famous line of Laurel and Hardy from the dark past when some of us were young. Eliza turned heel, picked up her purse and went out the door, thinking of this fine mess of her own, realizing that it was a mess she had to deal with... and soon.

Perhaps if she drove around for awhile, her mother might calm down. She thought about visiting Carla and reasoned that talking with the only person she knew of that was at all close to Alice might be a prudent move.

Carla saw Eliza's car come into the driveway and she went to meet the young woman. "How did it go, dear? Did you learn anything about your mother's condition?"

"I certainly did," Eliza replied. "I learned enough to realize that my problems have only just begun! I'm going to need your help ... and the help of anyone else you can think of!"

The two women went into Carla's inviting kitchen. Carla pulled out the cups, saying, "Coffee or tea?" "Or perhaps a new life?"

Eliza broke down into tears, sobbing about how her mother didn't even realize there was something wrong with her and that she had told her to get out of the house. She explained about the testing that Dr. G had done and that her mother really failed all the tests. She then told Carla about the extent of the planning that had to be done, wondering how she could ever get any of it completed.

Wisdom comes with age, so they tell me. Carla was truly a wise woman. She pointed out to Eliza that there were many people and agencies which could support her in her travels through the wonderland which had become Alice's life.

Carla herself had been through a similar circumstance when her father had a stroke, leaving her in charge of his life. Her mother had died many years ago. Fortunately, Carla had an older brother nearby whose strength she found most helpful during the hard weeks.

"First," Carla said to Eliza, "don't worry about your mother telling you to get out of the house. By the time we finish this coffee cake, she will have forgotten what she said."

"How is that possible," Eliza replied. "She was so angry, I just can't imagine her forgetting the mean things she said to me. I really don't know how I'm ever going to be able to find out about her financial affairs and legal things like the deed to the house, and a will, if she has one."

"Right now, Eliza, the main thing is that you take a deep breath, and we'll make a list of some of the things that need doing. This is just like what I went through with Dad when he was not able to take care of himself," Carla said, in a calm, relaxing voice.

"Let's make a list of what we know and what we need to know," Carla said. "You know now that your mother's previous physician has been deceased for about a decade. Whether or not someone or some firm has his medical records might be helpful, but I really doubt that we are going to learn anything on that score. At least we will have the report from Dr. G to use in case you have to go to court for a guardianship petition."

"Guardianship? You don't really think that will be necessary, do you?" Eliza replied. "I can't imagine that she would ever let me be her guardian, knowing how closed mouth she is about her affairs," said Eliza.

"And that's just the point," Carla added. "You won't have to wait for her to allow you to be a guardian; that will be the decision of the court. It all depends on her level of impairment. In order to have a guardian appointed, one must show that the person in question is incompetent to make decisions and unable to care for themselves in a safe manner," explained Carla.

They decided to place that particular situation at the bottom of their "to do" list. Other items came before that, and an important matter was settling up the financial mess which Alice had created by not paying bills. Carla suggested that Eliza make phone calls as soon as possible to all those waiting for payment.

"Where should I look to find the unpaid bills? asked Eliza. "I know about those that were on the kitchen table but there may be many others."

Carla smiled and said, "Knowing your mother, she probably has them in the top drawer of her dresser. I remember when your Dad was alive, she always kept important papers there. You might even find some clue as to her bank accounts, too," she commented.

"I hate to be snooping in her things but I guess that's the only way we're going to find out the true situation. I know Dad had an attorney who was a golfing buddy.

Do you suppose I could talk with him to see if there are legal papers I should know about?" Eliza seemed to be getting stronger and had a better grasp on the situation at hand.

By the time the coffee cake was gone and the coffee pot empty, Eliza and Carla had put together a rather lengthy list of 'chores' for the next day. Taking her leave, Eliza thanked Carla and said, "If you are right, Mom will have forgotten that I caused her trouble. We'll see how she's doing now."

The short trip to Alice's home gave Eliza a chance to put together the scenario of how she would handle her mother's mercurial behavior pattern.

"Where have you been?" asked Alice as Eliza came in the door. "I haven't seen you since we went to that woman's office."

Relieved that the tumultuous incident had been forgotten, Eliza smiled at her now docile mother saying, "I ran into an old friend and we got to talking. Would you like to go to your favorite restaurant for dinner?"

"That sounds lovely. Just wait until I comb my hair and we can leave." Alice turned to go to the powder room off the kitchen, saying, "You think of the nicest things, Eliza!"

And so we close this chapter of "Eliza Faces Life" wondering: "Will Alice behave in the restaurant? Will Eliza find the bank papers? Will she be able to get the unpaid bills? Will this ever end?"

OLLEY, OLLEY, ALL'S IN FREE!

Hide and seek, right? Oxen free, according to some people. I wonder if the kids of this generation know about that call?

Well, hide and seek certainly described Eliza's dilemma the next day. She awakened in what had been her room during her youth. But she had never awakened wondering who the mother would be when she went down for breakfast! Would she be the pleasant woman whom she had taken to dinner last night or would she be the vicious crone who told her to get out of the house? This was an entirely new situation and it appeared that there were no rules to this game. She guessed she would have to make up the rules as she went along, knowing that it would be fruitless to confront her mother in an adversarial way. Oh, boy. Fun today, no doubt!

Alice was sitting at the breakfast table with a perplexed look on her face.

"Did you know that I don't have to teach today?" she remarked. "I had a call from the Principal and she said that my class was going to be covered. Covered by what? What do you think she meant?"

49

Eliza stalled for time. "Let me get a cup of coffee and we'll talk about it," she replied. "I think I know what she meant. But wait … I think I'll make myself some toast, too."

Coffee cup in hand, Eliza faced her mother, dreading what she had to tell her.

"Mom," she started, "Remember when we went to see Dr. G yesterday and she asked you all those questions? Well, she was testing your memory to see if you could still remember things."

Alice interrupted, "But I have a fine memory. Didn't I do a great job on those tests?"

"Actually, no. Dr. G was trying to learn if your short term memory was still in tact. She knew you could remember certain things from many years ago but she was concerned that you had difficulty in some of the tests. This isn't your fault, Mom. This sometimes happens in people. It isn't caused by anything you did. It only means that there is a problem with your brain and we want to do everything we can to make your life as easy as possible," Eliza said. "And because we learned that you are having a problem, the Principal decided that she would get someone to take over your class for the rest of the year so that we can settle some of the problems."

Alice sat quietly, apparently stunned by what Eliza was telling her. "You mean I don't have to go into school at all for the remainder of the school year?

"That's right," said Eliza. "But we can talk about school later, now that you know that it is being taken care of for you. I'd like to help you with paying some bills I found here on the kitchen table. Can we look at them together?"

It must have been the good fates who were in charge of Alice's personality that morning for she agreed to go over those bills and several others she had stashed away in the top drawer of her dresser. Eliza had to smile when her mother went to the dresser, remembering what Carla had told her the previous day. Sure enough, there was quite a pile of envelopes, some opened but many still sealed.

"Let's look at these first," said Eliza, taking up the pile of opened envelopes. "Perhaps there are some duplicates here. Maybe some of those you haven't opened yet are the same as these in this stack," she said. Always maintaining a low tone of voice and a gentle smile, it would have appeared to a new comer that the two women were merely chatting about some innocent event in their future rather than attempting to learn the extent of the mess which had been created by the combination of memory loss and bills unpaid. Better to use honey than vinegar, as the old adage tells us.

Eliza soon found that there were certainly duplicates among the bills, but in most cases they were reminders of non-payment with added late charges and final notices which demanded payment. It was easy to see that this pile could be drastically cut by tossing out the bills from six months, four months, even two months ago. No duplication needed here!

Her next job was to carefully ask her mother where her checkbook was located so that she could start balancing the account prior to paying bills.

"Mom, can you tell me where you keep your check book? I think we might want to make sure everything is in balance before we pay these bills." Eliza knew that the low voice and simple talk seemed to be working and so she continued in that mode. (Don't rock the boat!)

You can see where this is going. When Eliza was given the check book, she found that not only had her mother not entered any checks written for over a year, she had no accounting of what monies were going in to the account. It seemed apparent to Eliza that this was going to take more than paying a few bills to get things straightened out. That was when she decided to bring up the question of a lawyer.

"Do you remember that nice lawyer who was Dad's friend? I think he helped you with Dad's estate after he died. Have you spoken with him lately?" queried Eliza.

"You mean Hi? Hiram was your father's golfing buddy, too. I haven't heard from him for quite a while. Why do you want to talk with him?" Alice asked.

"Well," Eliza replied, "I want to know about deposits to your account which would have come from Dad's retirement and from your teaching. I think we need to bring everything up to date to make it easier for you," she said, knowing that stressing the "easier for you" would go down better than "so we can take over your life."

Alice agreed and Eliza went to the phone to make an appointment with Atty. Hiram, for the earliest possible date.

Eliza couldn't get over how calm and reasonable her mother had been and only hoped that this stage would last until they had met with Hiram. She really didn't need to have the wicked witch from the west come back into play in the lawyer's office!

Later that afternoon, Eliza drove Alice downtown to Hiram's office. By the time they were seated in the conference room, and had gone through the usual opening banter of how are you and it's nice to see you again, Eliza started to explain to Hiram what she had learned of her mother's difficulties and of the meeting with Dr. G the previous day. All was well until Alice started her Jekyll and Hyde change. Was this the same woman who had been so easy to speak with over breakfast?

Alice was in fine form as she told Hiram, "I don't know what my daughter is talking about. She came home a little while ago and starting insisting that I wasn't doing things right and that my memory was gone and all sorts of horrible things were happening to me. I don't know why she is acting this way," she yelled, sobbing as she spoke.

Hiram was his old sedate self, having seen similar occurrences through the years he had been in practice. Dementia may not be easily recognized by some physicians but you can bet that lawyers who practice family law, including wills, guardianship, powers of attorney and the like, have seen it all. Families who have always been caring, easy going and solid in their appreciation and love for one another can suddenly become snarling, grabbing brats when the affairs of the infirmed parent are being discussed.

I mention this because many people believe that their family will always be close without turmoil or strife. Hmmmmm.

Once upon a time there was a family comprised of one father, one deceased mother and three offspring. When father was diagnosed with Alzheimer's disease, it was suddenly determined, without any discussion among the siblings, that the son living in the same town would be the person to care for Dad. The other siblings would be available "in a pinch" to help out. When it reached the point that Dad needed a guardian because he had progressed to end stage dementia, it brought the three adult children together, still in agreement that the male who had been the primary (?) caregiver would be named guardian. That was until the other two realized that it wasn't only the caregiving that guardianship would entail. Money came in to the picture and the green-eyed monster of jealousy reared up in the midst of the talks.

"What do you mean?" asked the eldest sister. "You are going to be in control of Dad's money and you plan to put him in a nursing home? Over my dead body will Dad ever be in a nursing home!"

To which the 'good son with the exhausted wife' replied, "We can't care for him any more. We are at the house every day and we take turns staying with him at night. We just can't do it anymore. Do either of you want to take care of him?"

[That particular story ended when the 'good son' refused to be the guardian, left the room, and did not speak to his siblings for over two years. The sibs, not wanting to devote their lives to caring for this shell of a man, put him in the nursing home and grouched about it for their remaining years.]

Back to the show at Hiram's office. When he realized the extent of Alice's dementia, he asked his assistant to draw up several documents, including a durable power of attorney, a health care proxy, a living will (should she ever be out of state when an advance directive was needed) and preliminary conservator ship papers. He then told Eliza that since he had been executor of her father's estate, he had all the information she was searching for and, in fact, had a statement of all the deposits which had been make to Alice's account as well as a listing of other financial holdings such as CDs and a portfolio of stocks which were being attended to by his office. While Alice had been informed of all these matters, it certainly appeared that she did not, as of this moment, remember those facts.

His suggestion to Eliza was that she continue to write checks for the outstanding bills, showing Alice what was being done and having Alice sign the checks. He also suggested that perhaps the morning hours might be better for this purpose since it appeared that her mother might be experiencing a "sundown syndrome" episode which often occurs later in the day in some dementia patients. It also might have been brought about by coming to his office… something which would, to Alice, be out of her usual routine schedule.

Alice had calmed down substantially by this time. However, Hiram thought that the signing of a power of attorney and other papers might be easier accomplished if he came by the house the next day, which was a Saturday. Eliza agreed and suggested that he come for lunch since she had already planned to cook one of her mother's favorites for the meal.

And so the curtain comes down once again on the continuing saga of "Life Can Be A Mess" knowing that there are many other pitfalls to be addressed tomorrow!

"Slowly She Turned, Inch by Inch ..."

T hank you, Google. I can never remember the sources of these weird phrases, so I have to depend on the giant data base of the offspring of Barney Google.

(For the younger crowd, say under age 50, Barney G. was a comic strip in antiquity.)

O. K. So that's not the real beginning of it, but it will have to do for now. Actually, I understand the phrase came from either an old Abbott & Costello flick or perhaps The Three Stooges. Once again, I digress.

Back at the old homestead, Alice was in her pleasant mode. She had been up early and cooked waffles for her daughter. To be truthful, she put a couple in the toaster. When Eliza first smelled the toaster, she thought something was amiss but was relieved to find that the only thing wrong was there were two black things burning. They could not be identified as waffles, but since they hadn't set the room afire, it was probably a near miss.

Which, of course, gave Eliza something else to worry about. Could her mother be left alone in this house with no one to check on her activities? That was a subject which had not come into her mind until that morning. She never thought of a fire. Or of her mother wandering away from the house. Or, driving off with no intention of becoming lost, but nevertheless ending up in the next State. Truly, this old scary cliché of "inch by inch, step by step" from the monster movies seemed to have taken over the whole enormous situation.

It was Saturday and Hiram was coming for lunch. Eliza decided to make a grocery shopping list to have food available for Alice. When she had glanced over the inside of the refrigerator the previous day, she had noted that there was a good supply of baking soda in the back, some plastic containers which might or might not have contained edible food (she really didn't want to look for fear that Alice was growing a colony of green or gray mold) and a freezer full of aluminum wrapped whatevers... which had no labels attached.

Alice was a light eater at breakfast, contrary to what she had told Dr. G the previous day. She really did like her coffee and appeared still able to make coffee in the automatic machine on the counter. If the toaster didn't stick, as it did with the waffles, she could be expected to make toast. Orange juice was in good supply in the refrigerator. When she was teaching every day, a noontime meal could be substantial enough to count as the main meal of the day. As for her evening meal, Eliza thought that her mother was probably skipping that event, either because there wasn't available food that was easy to prepare or because she just simply forgot. Alice did appear to have lost some weight … a loss she could ill afford since she was rail thin most of her life.

Another quandary: how do you find out whether or not the person is eating (correctly) or if they can still cook an easy meal? Eliza had heard stories the "tea and toast" ladies who ended up in the hospital with malnutrition and dehydration. She certainly didn't want that to happen to her mother. But, how to solve the problem… without turning Alice into that monster seen the previous day.

"Mom," Eliza asked, "where do you do your grocery shopping now? I see that there are several super markets in town. Do you go there or to the old local grocery store on the edge of town?"

"You ask the strangest questions, Eliza. Why would you care where I shop? Are you going to tell me I have to go somewhere else for food? What's the matter?" asked Alice.

Oops. It seems as if Mom is a bit testy this morning. Time to change the subject and go back to it later.

"Oh, nothing, Mom. I was just curious as to how the old store was doing with all the competition from the big chains." Another confrontation avoided.

With a quick change of subject, Eliza reminded her mother that Hiram was coming for lunch today and she had promised to make that salad that the family always liked. It was a depression era dish, but still popular with many folks. She asked Alice if there were apples in the house (knowing that none were in plain sight) and did she still keep chopped walnuts in the pantry.

Alice brightened when some of the salad ingredients were mentioned. "Yes, I do have some walnuts but I think we'll have to go out to the orchard to get the apples. I have some celery, I think. Do you need something else?"

Here was a perfect example of getting her mother involved in a small project which she knew could be completed with little difficulty. While Eliza knew there were no apples, she was also very much aware that no celery could be living in those hydrator drawers in the refrigerator. Good time to suggest a quick shopping trip.

It was a bit cool for the time of year so Eliza suggested her mother get a sweater to put on. This, too, was a chance to see how the clothing situation was and whether or not proper clothing was ready to wear… or were we still in the Capri pants and sleeveless blouse stage?

Alice appeared, purse in hand, wearing a flimsy summer dress and sandals. Eliza decided this was *not* the time to have a confrontation. She let the attire pass, thinking that if mother became chilly, there was a sweater in the back of Eliza's car.

Off to the orchards which were in the midst of the boom season with many locals and some from out-of-State taking the side roads to pick up the New England brands of apples. When the mother and daughter arrived, the parking lot was pretty full of cars but Alice seemed to enjoy the excitement of the smells and sights of the barn, full of baskets and bags of apples, pears, peaches and assorted drinks including cider freshly pressed and some local milk from the dairy close by. Alice looked happier than at any time since Eliza had first come home.

Many people with dementia have a special appreciation for places, things and events which remain in the memory because they have a special meaning for the impaired person. Some holiday or family events … things connected to their past, such as their appreciation of nature or of the fruits and vegetables of the local geographic area. It may be different with each section of the country, but most caregivers have found that it is the simple things which often give the greatest pleasure to those whose cognitive abilities have been damaged.

Alice remembered the name of the fellow who was taking the money and bagging the purchases. His grandfather had tended the orchards many years ago and the young man who was in charge today had been one of Alice's students some thirty years previous.

Apples placed in the back seat, they were off to pick up lettuce, mayonnaise, more nuts, celery and a few white grapes as well as raisins to add to the salad. All through this next stop, Alice seemed a bit quiet. The super market might have been too overwhelming for her. Large crowds can be upsetting as too much stimulation produces anxiety in some people with this type of brain disorder. Soon they were back home. Eliza washed vegetables and apples while Alice easily peeled and chopped the fruit. Some familiar tasks remain with us many years after the higher levels of cognition have failed.

While Eliza put the finishing touches on the Waldorf salad, warmed rolls and made iced tea, Alice decided to use her linen bridge tablecloth with the matching napkins. It was her decision to put the small bowl of African violets in the center of the table as a special touch.

When Hiram arrived, he was pleasantly surprised to see a lovely table setting, calm people and good food awaiting him. Any 'shop talk' would be left until after dessert.

But that time came quickly; it was time to discuss legal matters and to do it in the quietest, easiest way possible. The fact that Hiram and Alice's husband had been good friends made the chore much easier on all concerned.

Hiram talked with Alice about the state of her personal legal and financial affairs. Alice listened quietly, not questioning any of the material. He explained how the deposits from her husband's retirement were being transferred directly into her account without any individual help from her. He also told Eliza that he had filed her mother's income taxes every year after Alice had seen them and signed the forms. The fact that Alice didn't seem to remember any of this was not of importance, particularly as it was not upsetting to her and was being done in a legally acceptable manner.

When he brought up the need to have a durable power of attorney in force, he was extremely careful to explain exactly what this paper would do for her in case she was not able to handle matters for herself. After his explanation, he asked her if she understood what he had said. She replied that she could understand why this was needed, although she didn't believe it would ever be necessary to use the document. As long as she was able to understand the document, and appeared to be cognizant and aware of what she was doing, Hiram had Alice sign the paper.

Note: As long as she knew, *at that particular time*, what she was doing, this would be legal. Everyone should check their own State laws.

Alice's will had been signed several years before and there did not seem to be reason to make any changes to that document.

The Massachusetts Health Care Proxy allows an individual over eighteen years of age to sign a form designating that the chosen person named in the document has been given the right to make healthcare decisions for the primary person in case that person in unable to make those decisions for any number of reasons, including coma, trauma, stroke, dementia, or many other instances. An attorney is not needed to make such a document and most if not all hospitals have blank forms which an individual may fill out. The document does require that it be signed in front of two witnesses; a notary public is NOT needed.

Eliza explained to her mother that she, herself, had such a document and showed her mother the card that she carried with her at all times. She also told Alice that a copy of her document was at the local hospital, in her doctor's files and in her attorney's files as well as in her home where her private papers are kept.

Alice's good mood seemed to have been maintained; was it the Waldorf salad?

"Yes," she said, shaking her head in affirmation, "That seems to be a good thing to do. I remember when your Dad died, I had to make all kinds of decisions. We didn't have that kind of paper then, did we?"

Hiram smiled and told her, "You were there, Allie, and I knew you would do what he would want." End of another problem.

"You know, Alice," Hiram added, "I think it might be a good idea to have Eliza's name added to your checking account and other financial papers. It's always wise to have someone who can check on things for you when you want answers."

Smoothie that he was, Alice was beaming under the attention and agreed with whatever he had to offer. Good thing that Eliza knew he was an honest man as well as a fine attorney and a good friend.

Lunch over, it was time for Hiram's departure and a nap for Alice. I wouldn't have been surprised if Eliza, too, didn't "rest her eyes" a bit!

THE PLOT THICKENS
(OR IS THAT 'A WATCHED POT WON'T BOIL'?)

E liza knew that the calm, serene Alice couldn't be counted on to remain in place. Everything was too copacetic. Nothing like getting up in the morning and knowing where you are but having no idea as to what people and events would face you this day.

The medical part of the problem had been addressed to some degree and the legal and financial picture was starting to come together. Her head swirling with thoughts of other matters that needed her attention, she was up early and had started breakfast before Alice was out of bed. Now *there's* a change in roles. Alice had always been up before first light in the past. Perhaps it was a sign that she was becoming more comfortable with the idea of being a retired teacher.

While the coffee perked or dripped or whatever it did, Eliza grabbed a legal pad she had picked up on their shopping trip and started making a list of chores that needed to be done, of situations that needed to be looked into and questions that needed answers.

First: Get back to Dr. G and ask for some guidance concerning her mother's ability to remain in her home without supervision. That reminded Eliza that she should probably ask about some of the medications she had heard about from friends at the hospital. She hoped that these might give Alice added time to make plans for the future.

Second: Find out about a support group for caregivers of family members with some form of dementia. Maybe the Alzheimer's Association could help with that. How can they be reached? Eliza tried the phone book, to no avail. Not in the white pages and not under any suspect groups in the yellow pages. What's this all about! *[As this chapter was written, I was in contact with the Mass. Alzheimer's Association office in Springfield where they learned, to their surprise, that they had been omitted. By the time this book is in print, I'm certain you will find the proper telephone number.]*

Good old internet: Alzheimer's Association web page with all sorts of connections and more help than Eliza could have imagined!

The next stage to be conquered was what to do about the license to drive the car. Although Eliza knew of at least two events involving problems with driving, she wanted to have something more concrete in her cache of information. Remembering something a colleague had told her while at work at the hospital, she began looking for a neuropsychologist who practiced in the area. She also put in a call to Dr. G to see if she had someone to whom she referred patients in need of this type of examination. Indeed she did! With name, address and phone number in hand, she called to make an appointment for Alice. Fortunately, there was a cancellation that very afternoon if she could get her mother there.

Eliza called Dr. G's office, requesting that she fax the basic information to Dr. Jaye, the neuropsychologist. Now if Alice was in one of her better personas, the big test was set to go.

Neuropsychological testing is not new but it certainly took a huge jump in recognition by the general public with the increase in the number of persons being diagnosed with some form of dementia. This form of testing involves a series of rather simple tests which include remembering words, recognizing pictures shown and repeated, spatial testing, putting puzzle pieces together, asking the client to name objects placed before them and often, the clock face test mentioned previously.

Because this type of test has been used worldwide for decades now, there is a large body of data indicating that certain errors indicate damage to the corresponding part of the brain. Some patients appear quite normal until they undergo this form of testing. Some people who haven't had an accident while driving may learn that the part of their brain which controls judgment (among other things) has been damaged and that their ability to recognize dangerous driving situations such as a sign that a bridge is out, may not be able to process that information to avoid an accident. Too, the part of the brain that allows us to remember the route we wish to take and the ability to recognize certain landmarks may not be functioning properly. Have you heard stories about people driving away from home and then being found in the next State? Often the impaired person seems competent to drive yet neuropsychological testing may indicate that this is an extremely dangerous situation and that the person so impaired should stop driving immediately.

Eliza knew in her heart that this would probably be the case with her mother but she also knew that a battle was brewing ahead should this information come out in the doctor's report.

Here's a story told to me by a colleague in another State.

Alonzo Kay lived alone in a single family home in the outskirts of a Town in rural New York. His wife had died some ten years before and he had managed fairly well to keep the house (and himself) in respectable condition. As he approached his 78th birthday, he was finding it difficult to remember things... like his own telephone number, the grocery items he needed, his appointments, and even the location of his three children.

When his third broken appointment with his physician occurred, the office tried to reach him, to no avail. Dr. L. decided that something was definitely amiss and put in a call to the emergency contact on Mr. Kay's record... his son, Mac, who lived in Syracuse.

Mac was at home when Dr. L. called. He was unaware that his father had any problems; he had seemed fine when the family was last together for the 4th of July. It was now early October and Mac admitted that his only contact with his father had been by phone once a week. He told Dr. L that he would be in touch with his two siblings and they would be at their Dad's home the following Friday afternoon. Dr. L told Mac he would set up an appointment for 4:30 that afternoon so that they could all get together and discuss the situation.

Mac called his older brother, Nat, and his younger sister, Olive, to give them the news and to ask that they meet the following Friday afternoon at the office of Dr. L. Mac would pick up his father and take him to the meeting.

Mac was sure he could relax for a day or two before facing his father, something he was dreading because of the father's history of rejecting any help from the kids.

Sure enough, just as he decided he had a reprieve for a day or two, the phone rang. It was the local police in the Town where his father resided, telling him that his father had been picked up and was at the station. "We'll talk about the incident when you get here," said the Desk Officer.

Wondering what could have happened to his father that would involve the local police, Mac jumped into his car and drove immediately to the station. When he entered the front door, he could hear his father's voice, stridently informing the officer that he had done nothing wrong.

"Hi, Dad," said Mac, hoping that his presence would somehow deflate the anger he heard in his father's voice. "What seems to be the matter here?" he asked. The young officer showed Mac to a chair, remarking, "Your Dad had a small mishap this afternoon as he was entering the southbound ramp on Route 5, but he drove up the exit ramp instead of the entrance."

Mr. Kay became agitated, yelling at the officer, "They must have moved the road; I've always gone that way. You didn't see the signs right." To which the young officer replied, quite politely, "I'm sorry sir, but you were at fault." And to Mac, he added, "This isn't the first time we've had a problem with your father. A few weeks ago he came out of a restaurant parking lot and made a left turn into oncoming traffic. We didn't press charges at the time because your father told us he was going to be moving away and wouldn't be in this area any more."

Dumbfounded didn't really describe this "Alice In Wonderland" episode. Mac shook his head, trying to discern the extent of the problem and tease out which parts made sense and which were pure fabrication. He was sure of one thing; his father was in the wrong and the police were correct.

After explaining to the police that his father had recently been diagnosed with a memory problem, he asked the officer what charges would be made against his Dad. "Let me say first, I plan to stay with my Dad for the rest of the week and I can guarantee that he will not be driving. In fact, I believe that when we have seen all the medical people necessary, he will no longer have a license," Mac said.

Mr. Kay stared at his son and said, "What do you mean I'm not going to drive? I have been a good driver all my life. Why should I stop now?"

The officer could see that this problem would no longer be one which the police would have to handle and said to Mac, "I think we can safely say that this event will be presented to the Court as a misdemeanor to be handled by the family. Why don't you take your Dad home and we'll be in touch with you later."

Mac and his father left the station in Mac's car. His father was very angry with his son and didn't understand why he was being punished.

"You said you were going to stay with me for the rest of the week? You never told me that. Why are you here?" he said to his son.

"Let's wait until we get home, Dad. Things are going to be all right."

So Mac called his wife back in Syracuse and then called Nat and Olive to let them know the current status. The two agreed to come to their father's home on Friday morning so that they could have a talk with Dad before the meeting with the doctor.

The outcome in this event was that Mr. Kay was found to have mid-stage dementia, probably of the Alzheimer's type. Because he tested at mid-stage, Dr. L advised the family to (1) remove the car and dispose of it in whatever manner would work best to the advantage of all. He also suggested that Mr. Kay's license be returned to the New York Motor Vehicle Registry, along with a letter from Dr. L stating that Mr. Kay was incompetent to be on the road.

Incompetence is a legal term and laws vary from State to State. In this particular case, all involved were in accord that Mr. Kay was not competent to drive.

Dr. L then described to the family the problems involved in allowing their father to continue to live alone, particularly since he could no longer care for himself. The crux of this problem was the safety of Mr.

Kay. He had already demonstrated that his judgment was impaired, that his memory was fallible and his ability to remain in the current situation would put his life at risk.

Mr. Kaye moved to Syracuse and stayed with his son, Mac and his wife. Attending an Adult Day Health program sponsored by the Council on Aging; he remained with them until he fell one day, fracturing his hip. Following surgery, he moved to a local rehabilitation facility which had a special wing for residents with forms of memory impairment.

So you see, it was really a fortuitous automotive event which brought the family together to care for their father. Would a similar event be the answer to Alice's problems? That was what Eliza was thinking

I guess those old commercials about waking up and smelling the coffee have a grain of truth. It wasn't but a quarter of an hour later that Alice could be heard puttering around upstairs. That was the sign for Eliza to push the lever on the toaster; she really knew her mother's day to day routine.

"What are you doing?" asked Alice, taking her seat by the window. "What's that scribbling on the pad about?"

Eliza brought her mother juice, a cup of coffee and toast, ready for her choice of butter, jam or cinnamon sugar.

"I was starting a list of things we probably should do while I'm here," said Eliza. She was hoping that use of the word "we" might let her get through the most difficult parts of the list.

"What kind of things," Alice said, a suspicious look coming on to her face. "Are you planning to put me in a nursing home? I won't go, you know. I'm perfectly happy where I am and I can take care of myself without anyone's help. I always have and I always will!"

"No, Mom, this has nothing to do with a nursing home. I'm just trying to pull my thoughts together so that you and I can talk about some things," Eliza replied. "Nothing so drastic as a nursing home. Besides, you have many good years ahead of you. We just want to be sure that you're safe as well as happy."

Alice's attention turned to the birds clamoring at the feeder in the yard. Eliza took the pause and refilled her coffee cup, thinking how to best tell Alice what needed to be done.

"Mom," she said, quite tentatively, "I spoke with Dr. G a bit ago. She would like you to see someone this afternoon. This is a different kind of doctor… one that will have you do some of the things your students did at school. She will have you put some pieces of a puzzle together, perhaps ask you to describe a picture, remember a grocery list… things like that."

Alice looked at her daughter, scowling at her as she described the testing procedure. "Just what are they going to learn from that rubbish?" she asked.

"Oh, come on, now… you know you always loved to take those tests in the women's magazines asking which color you'd pick or which menu sounded best! These are kind of like those except they will help us plan how you will be cared for in future years," Eliza said. She hoped that glossing over the neuropsychological testing would make her mother more amenable to going to see this psychologist.

Alice perked up a bit, sensing that this new thingamabob doctor might be o.k. after all.

They drove to Dr. Jaye's office in the early part of the afternoon. The waiting room was tastefully decorated in soothing colors, no jarring effect evident. The social worker who was doing the intake asked Alice a few simple questions and then led her to Dr. Jaye's office where the young woman greeted her with a smile and "I'm Dr. Jaye. I'm so glad you could come to see me today."

The social worker returned to Eliza, pointing to an adjoining room where the two women could talk and where Alice's history could be completed.

Eliza knew that the testing would probably take several hours and that Alice would be given a break between testing for some juice and perhaps a cookie or two. She also knew that the report wouldn't be available for a number of days. And knowing that, she told the social worker that since she was an only child and did not live in the immediate area, it was of utmost importance that she have *some* clue as to the status of her mother, vis a vis her ability to remain in her home with no other person living there.

The social worker eased by the question but did offer this: "Each person is different and each has a support system unique to their situation. Unless there are obvious deficits which would negate her staying in her home, it may be possible to make use of agencies in this area which can support her desire to remain independent."

Not exactly the answer Eliza was hoping to hear, but if that was all she could learn today, she had better put on her thinking cap and find out what was available from those agencies.

To Every Thing There is a Season?

It's amazing what can be done in a week's time when you are under great pressure to get things done. In addition to realizing that she was faced with almost insurmountable but necessary chores, Eliza also became aware that the holiday season was nearly upon her. She had only two more days to get all the pieces in place so that she could return home for the brief respite of going back to work!

Eliza was particularly fortunate to have three good people on board to assist in the care plan that had been drawn up for her mother's needs. Carla was what Alice had called a "shining light" in her life. Her dear friend had agreed to be the surrogate caregiver, working with the care manager and with Atty. Hiram. Now we would see if this carefully orchestrated plan would fly. (Do we have a mix of words here? Do flying and orchestration complement each other? Who cares!)

As she packed to return home to her family, Eliza checked once again with all those involved to be sure they were all following the same game plan... or is it that they all had to be "on the same page"?

Dementia, in whatever form it takes, is fraught with ups and downs, good days and bad, and symptoms which occur frequently with some people and never in others. In this case, we had already seen fluctuations in mood in Alice, as well as large holes in her recent memory. By observing her in her day to day life, Eliza had been able to pinpoint problems which were already obvious and she had also found that there were other inconsistencies in her behavior which she had not attributed to dementia... but, in fact, were 'dementia in action'.

It was time to go. How would Alice take her departure?

The Saturday morning when Eliza planned to leave was miserable with typical late fall drizzle, winds out of the northwest, and a dreariness in the landscape caused by the first killing frost which had occurred during the past two days.

Alice was in the kitchen when Eliza came down, laden with suitcase, duffle bag and pocketbook.

"Are you going somewhere, dear?" asked Alice. "Did you tell me you were leaving? I don't seem to remember things very well these days. Where are you going?" she asked.

Eliza thought of the talk she had with the care manager about carefully wording responses so as to keep the impaired person as calm as possible.

"Good morning, Mom. That coffee smells wonderful. You always made the very best coffee in the world." Calm voice, smiling face, careful words. How would Alice react?

"Sit down, dear. The coffee just finished and there are scones on the table. I think you bought them for me. Let's have a nice breakfast."

Had Alice forgotten her question about Eliza leaving? For the moment, it was in the back corridors of her mind. Breakfast was on the agenda and all was well in her world.

Sure that Alice was stable, Eliza broached the subject of her departure. "Last night when we had dinner with Carla, we talked about my need to go home to my family. The kids are still in school during the day but it's been hard for my husband, Ed, to run the house, the kids and his own work. I think you told me that we should be planning to come here for Thanksgiving with you. Do you remember our talking about that?"

"Oh, yes. And Carla told me that Halloween was next week. It doesn't seem possible that so much time has passed. We did talk about Thanksgiving, didn't we. It will be good to have all the family here. What are your children's names?"

That was a shock to Eliza, but she managed to gloss over it. "Ally is named for you, Mom, and Eddie is named for his father. Here... let me leave these pictures for you. I'll put them right here on the refrigerator so that you will see them every time you open the door!" Eliza thought she had handled that pretty well.

Just as she was starting to put her baggage in the trunk of her car, Carla arrived, with the new homemaker in tow. Her name was Terry, and she would help Alice with the laundry and then take her shopping in her car.

Alice's car had been taken to the garage and was being serviced and spruced up before being put on the market. Although Alice had given up her license, there would probably be times when she would not remember that her license was no longer in effect nor would she remember that the car is no longer available to her.

There was nothing else Eliza could do. She packed the car, kissed her mother good bye and started for home.

How long would it be before the telephone started ringing? How long would it be that Alice could live in her own home?

That's the problem with dementia; you can never count on life following a normal path. But Eliza realized that this past week of torment, feeling inadequate, not knowing what to do was just the beginning.

We leave Alice at home and Eliza driving home. Later in this book we'll take a look at how things are going with Alice. You know, of course, that there is much to come in their story!

Before we get into the series of cases covering just about everything you could possibly want to avoid, let me tell you how Alzheimer's became...

"OLD TIMER'S DISEASE"

They call it "Old timer's disease"

It is not my nature to criticize the way people pronounce certain words. I may bite my tongue, dying to speak, but generally I let it go. Things like "libRary" or "FebRuary" top the list, I think. When I hear commentators on television speak of something like the "LibAry of Congress" or an event to take place in "FebUary" I wonder, "Where have all the purists gone?"

Speaking at a Grange meeting several years ago, one of the farmers asked me if *Old timer's disease* was like getting hardening of the arteries. I knew then and there that we needed to 'spell' things out for these folks.

We've spoken about senility and becoming senile. But let's call a spade a spade and forego the niceties of verbiage.

The word is **DEMENTIA**. It has a distinct meaning and it refers to the ability of the brain to function in various modes of action. In other words, (Oh dear, it must be a Sinatra song), your brain stops working up to speed because of at least three distinct things: Thing One (thank you, Theodor Suess Geisel) is a loss of at least one of those chemicals that lets brain cells communicate. Thing Two is guck called Aβ or beta-amyloid which spends a lot of its time acting like a barnacle on the hull of a ship: it hangs on and finally kills the cell, with help from Thing Three which also has a Greek name … τ … pronounced 'tau' or even better, *taoow*

While the amyloid is on the outside, the tau is on the inside of the cell, doing a job on those ladders (known as microtubules) that hold together the twisted pieces of DNA. Mr. Inside (τ) is breaking up the DNA framework. Think of the tau segment as the rungs of that ladder. You've seen pictures of DNA with the pretty colors of the basic building blocks… guess what? They don't appear in living color in living life. Sorry about that. But τ does a great job of tearing down the ladder.

So… we have a chemical that needs a transfusion so that cells can talk to each other. We need Mr. Clean or one of similar bent who can dissolve that gunk called amyloid (or perhaps *stop* the stuff from forming there in the first place?) and we must find a way to send tau back where it came from. I don't think the Greeks would take it, however.

Now this is mid-2006, so don't hold me to this as being the 'end all' on that score. I know there are a dozen or more other aspects of the cause(s) of dementia of the Alzheimer's type just from reading the overwhelming tsunami of research from the Alzheimer's Research Forum, the various scientific publications and that word of mouth phenomenon which occurs with each conference, seminar or class attended.

Phenomenon? Reminds me of that old Muppets song **"men om men a"** which just goes to prove my eclectic interests. Either that or I spent too much time with my kids from Captain Kangaroo through Sesame Street, the Muppets and other great teaching media.

Let's get serious here, woman.

What happens with all these Things? Well, early scientists looked at the fact that a certain chemical, acetylcholine, was pretty scarce in the autopsied brains of people who had Alzheimer's. That's a very important chemical and when it gets to the point when you have only about 10% of it left in your brain, things aren't doing well at all. Cells can't communicate. Memories can't get encoded and sent on to the correct filing system part of the memory banks. (You must have noticed that most people with Alzheimer's have a pretty good memory about things that happened 40 or 50 years ago but sometimes they can't recognize their own daughter.)

Old memory banks are safe, at least for awhile. Medium banks may not be so hot, depending on how long this dementia thing has been going on, and recent banks are screwed. Oh, dear. Not a good term. Well, you get my message.

How come? Well, if the communication juice isn't there for the cells to get their message across, "Houston... we've got a problem." And if this happens say, some one or two million times a second, and the message that was <u>supposed</u> to be encoded and sent to the correct storage place **didn't**, then, whoops, no memory! If the input hits a stone wall and can't go anywhere, it just stays in the outer spaces of our mind. Never gets to our memory storage center. Got that?

Here's an easy one. You told your father that his brother called by telephone while he was out. He was looking right at you when you gave him the message. He smiled at you. He went back to looking out the window. Three hours later his brother calls again. You give your father the phone. His brother says to him, "Why didn't you call me back? I called you three hours ago." Your father looks at you and says, "Why didn't you tell me my brother called?"

AAAAGGGGGGGHHHHHH! (You may substitute Charlie Brown's favorite line!)

Maddening, isn't it? But that's what happens when the memory can't be encoded. You could have repeated your message to your father five minutes after the first conversation and the result would have been the same.

Back to those known causes of dementia. Bad enough we can't get the chemical up to speed, we've got that Aβ stuff that is gumming up the outside of the cells. Think of it this way: you're inside Capt. Nemo's submarine (Jules Verne type) and watching out for another sub, when you see slimy junk outside the porthole. No windshield wipers here. The unsightly gunk is forming on the whole window, cutting off the ability of the sub to do its work.

As if the Captain doesn't have enough problems, now the innards of the sub are being dissolved by some creature left over from a B movie of the 1940s. How long can it be before the sub is enveloped by the gunk and being dissolved by *whatever*!

Got the picture? Now put the whole thing in the brain. Let's start by attacking the area where the processing of memories starts. It's also the emotional center of the brain. If you see the words "hippocampus" and "frontotemporal lobe" or a reference to "medial temporal" area, don't panic. Your physician can explain those parts of the brain which are affected by this form of dementia. When those brain cells (which make up the parts described) are being attacked by the amyloid and tau enemies finally succumb, the whole part doesn't work. It's not like you can get along when only a few cells are involved. It's like that notorious 'flesh-eating bacteria' often seen in the news. Before you know it, too many parts are killed and the whole can not stand without the underpinnings which make up the organ.

You can see now why the various parts of the brain, some of which are in command of memory, others hold the keys to language, while others still are the leader: the frontotemporal area which forms judgment, sequential actions and other extremely necessary parts of the brain.

This might be a good place to talk about the **AAAA**s of Alzheimers. Actually they are symptoms of dementia, but we'll go with the *leading cause* of dementia: Alzheimers. They are better known as the cognitive function fellows. These are symptoms of brain problems, probably due to dementia, which are found deficient in **Agnosia** or changes in perception. This may be the cause of your husband saying to you, "Who are you?" The senses are getting information but the brain can't put it together right.

Aphasia, or language problems, may be expressive or receptive. It has a great many manifestations in addition to those mentioned here. It may be as simple as trying to find the right word. In dementia, the word *does not come back to you.* How about this: In late June, before July sets in, the CATALPA trees flower with their creamy white blossoms forming an upright bouquet on the end of the branches. They look similar to chestnut trees in leaf and bloom. A few weeks ago, I had a problem remembering the name of this tree. Was this a part of normal aging? Was it lack of concentration? Was I looking at the start of dementia? Nope. Just a glitch in the memory bank. Otherwise, how could I be telling you about it in this book?

Then there was the very intelligent woman who used to read four or five books every week. As her brain damage progressed, she would still have the books close at hand. However, reading and remembering what you have read means having an intact brain. The more intelligent the individual, the more educated, the easier it is to fool people into thinking the person is still capable of reading. Aphasia comes in all shapes and sizes!

Receptive aphasia is another ballgame altogether. What an impaired person hears is a jumble of sounds as though they had a hearing aid with a loose wire. Scratchy sounds that one can't control by tuning in to the right number on the FM dial.

Then we have the "Robin Hood's Barn" situation. *[I had to Google that one to be sure I had it spelled correctly. It means going the long way around to get to a place which, by direct route, would not have taken as long.]* In the case of those with a degree of aphasia, it may look like 'circumlocution' but the word I like better is the one used in referring to addition behavior… confabulation. They aren't exactly alike, but you will soon understand.

Maude is telling you that she would like a spoon to put sugar in her tea. She tells you, "Could I please have a…. a…. (she is now gesturing, too) a thing… to put in the (pointing) "… so it goes.   End of attempt. Fortunately, her use of gestures tells you a spoon is needed.

Maude's sister says, "I needed to pick up the…. you know, those things we saw last week when we went to the… then I came home and I knew I had done it right. Nothing. If this were an alcoholic, the confabulation would be to explain a black out and might sound something like "after I had a few drinks, I went to…. you know… down by the… Nuts. I knew I would get home because my buddy had his car and he took me." Similar, but not the same.

Amnesia is something you all have heard of, I'm sure. This is *not* the plot of a TV show. This is real. It means difficulty in learning new things. It may be either short or long term. Having been hit on the head in an automobile accident may cause a short term amnesia. Having lost parts of your memory encoding faculties will cause long term amnesia… meaning the same as your brother's telephone call that never got into the memory banks in the first place.

Apraxia, or decreased motor function. Better yet, the Dastoor-Mohr description in Gauthier's *Clinical Diagnosis and Management of Alzheimer's Disease:*

"ability to perform certain movements on demand, verbal command and on imitation."

In this case, the demented individual cannot do as requested, even though the muscles, bones, and **other physical parts are physiologically intact**. The person may be able to tell you what he/she has been asked to do, but the part of the brain that tells that part of the body what to do isn't connected.

I seem to be having that very problem. Not me, per se. It's my computer. I tell the computer to go to a certain internet site. I click on the proper site. Nothing happens. The computer (which I suspect has it in for me) is receiving electricity, is able to do some automatic things like booting up, but when I "tell it" to give me certain information, it suddenly becomes **apraxic** and refuses (or is it that, because of some internal damage, it cannot do it?) to do as asked. Got it?

Modern machinery. Marvelous. I still prefer a pen that works and plain paper, but should I attempt that combination, the printer would throw up his hands in frustration.

You tell Granny to sit down in this chair. You lead her to the chair. You repeat the request. Nothing. You try to show her what you want by sitting in the chair next to her. Nothing. Every muscle in her body is ready, but the brain isn't sending them a message.

So there we have: **Agnosia, Amnesia, Aphasia and Apraxia.**

Some have asked whether all the senses are damaged by dementia. The answer is yes and no. While the thinking part of the brain is damaged, other senses may be only marginally changed. For example, many have noted that a decrease in the sense of smell can be kind of an early warning sign of dementia. This may or not be true. There may be a problem with touch. By that I mean that if an impaired person were to reach into a bag containing several familiar objects, i.e. a comb, a spoon, a pen or pencil, that person might not be able to put a name to the object inside the bag and, at the same time, realize that it is indeed a familiar object. But what? Another example of agnosia at work.

It was thought for many years that sight was unharmed by dementia. I often wondered about that, particularly when I came in contact with many patients who insisted that someone had taken their glasses and left someone else's with them. I know that ophthalmologists are aware that caregivers often take their loved one for an appointment only to learn that there is no need for a prescription change. It isn't the glasses... it's the eyes. And not the usual problems, either. We now know that there is a change in the ability of the eye to transfer information via the optic nerve to the occipital (back) lobe of the brain. Much recent research also points to the inability of dementia patients to discriminate between light and dark areas, particularly if there is not an abundance of light. Lighting all areas of the living quarters may not only help the impaired person to recognize steps, carpets, and even eating utensils, it may help cut down on what has been known as 'sundown syndrome' (even when the sun isn't down). We know that some falls which have been attributed to rugs on floors, balance problems, even too much medication, might truly be charged up to dimming of the eyesight. Remember, this is not what the healthy adult might say was pure clumsiness. The sight in the patient with Alzheimer's can't see clearly and no trips to have the glasses changed will help. It's not cataracts. It's not glaucoma. It's not macular degeneration. We may not have a name for it right now, but let's just remember that bright lights, at all times, is the best thing you can do to keep your loved one more aware of surroundings. **BRIGHT LIGHTS**. You'll remember that!

There is another problem which might seem to be in the same venue as what was last described. It usually happens to patients in the mid to late stages of dementia and is not something which is universal to all patients. It's called the capgras syndrome.

Capgras syndrome may be responsible for some of the saddest stories. I have had wives come to a support group meeting in tears because their impaired husband told them he "didn't know who they were" and "what did you do with my wife?"

While this may appear to be purely a case of agnosia, there is a slight difference. In other cases, when the daughter is the caregiver, the father may make inappropriate sexual overtures, believing that the daughter is in fact his wife. I know this is hard to explain; it's hard for families to accept!

One daughter told a story about her mother who lived with her second husband in a small town west of here. The mother was in her 70s when this occurred. The mother's husband, a good, kind man, was redecorating their house when his wife was diagnosed with dementia, probably resulting from oxygen deprivation during a surgical procedure some years previous. The husband continued with his work, wanting to have everything in order so that he could care for his wife without having to 'fix this' or 'change that' to their home. His intentions were good.

One change in the house was a full length closet in the bedroom. There were folding doors to make everything neat and plenty of room for all types of clothes. All seemed to be going well until he realized that his wife didn't want to go into the room. She would quietly whisper, "Don't bother her. What's she doing there? I don't want her here!"

At first he was completely baffled. Then one day he found his wife with a plate of peanut butter crackers. He followed her at a distance and watched her go into the bedroom. She stayed as close to the wall as possible, sneaking up on the closet. When she was ready, she bent down, opened the door a few inches at the bottom, and snuck the snack inside. Then she left the room.

Fortunately, the daughter (who told me the story) was also a Gerontological nurse who specialized in respite care in an adult day health program. When her stepfather told her about the incident, she knew exactly what the problem was and how to fix it. "Take all those mirrors off the closet doors! She doesn't recognize her own reflection and she believes there is someone living in that room behind the mirrored doors."

How did she happen to pick up on this so quickly? There had been a woman at the day program who wouldn't go in the bathroom because there was a woman peeking at her. It was the mirror. So remember, the capgras syndrome has many faces.

Alison was another woman who was deeply troubled by her husband's reaction to her. They had been married nearly fifty years and had been together constantly during all that time. One day about five years after her husband had been diagnosed with Alzheimer's disease, he called out to her. "Ally … come in here. I need you." He was seated in the living room, relaxing in his recliner.

"What is it dear," she said, expecting that something must be terribly wrong from the tone of his voice.

"No. You're not Ally. Where's the other Ally? You get out of here. What have you done with her!" His anxiety was becoming very obvious. Ally left the room, hoping that her absence would allow him to somehow put these two Allys together.

As much as we would like to say that this is a rare occurrence, it wouldn't be quite true. Some have described events during which the man or woman became anxious because of the inability to recognize the person before them while still seeing a younger version of the same person. It would seem that some patients with dementia are looking through an old fashioned stereopticon viewer which should bring the two pictures together to form a   3-D effect yet, because of the brain damage, both pictures of the same person cannot merge. The events usually pass and the impaired person can once again see that the husband, now 75, is the same person as the 35 year old in "the mind's eye."

While we are looking at some of the behaviors most distressing to families, we should mention two other events… not capgras (or crap gas as one man described it) yet certainly in the "delusions and hallucinations" difficulty.

Alex was a man in his late 60s, living with his wife and two adult children in a town in southern Vermont. He had been a police officer during his working years and had been diagnosed at one of the testing facilities at the Medical Center of Southwestern Vermont. He had a thorough physical examination including a series of neuropsychological tests which indicated that he did indeed have dementia and that he might be prone to experiencing hallucinatory episodes.

The rule of thumb for many years has been that if the hallucination is not bothering the patient or those around him/her, leave it alone … don't treat with antipsychotic drugs, if at all possible. On the other hand, if the "vision" is causing great anxiety and distress, it may be time to make use of some of the newer medications designed for this type of event.

Alex's family were all living at home after Alex was diagnosed with Alzheimer's and all had become aware of a degree of suspiciousness not seen before. While paranoia and behaviors indicating that the person is being suspicious without cause are often seen in midstage dementia, what Alex's sons were seeing was very out of the ordinary in their formerly open, gregarious father. Their mother, too, couldn't understand what was going on with her husband.

One late afternoon, Josh, the older son, found his father out in the garage, cleaning a hunting rifle.

Fair warning here: It there are firearms of any sort in or around your household and there is an impaired person living in the house, PLEASE remove all such items. If

you insist on keeping some of these weapons, at least move them to the home of a friend who will be willing to keep them safe for you. NEVER have a firearm in the same house as a dementia patient.

Not wanting to create a scene with his Dad, Josh simply said, "Dad, I think Mom has been calling for you. Why don't you go in and find her." For once, Josh hoped that the dementia would not allow his father to remember the message.

While Alex walked to the house, Josh took the rifle apart, removed all ammunition, and also picked up two other guns in the garage. They were quickly sequestered in the trunk of Josh's car.

Returning to the kitchen, Josh noticed that Alex had gone into the front hall closet. "Mom," he whispered, "I got rid of all of Dad's guns out in the garage. They're in the trunk of my car, for now." "If he tells you that you were looking for him, just tell him you found what you were looking for!"

Later that night, Josh and his brother, Jed, came home around midnight. They were in Jed's car and he pulled in next to his brother's car. As they were getting out of the car, Jed stopped, looked around, and said in a whisper to his brother, "Do you hear someone walking around behind the house?"

"Yeah," said Josh. Someone is running, then stopping. Grab your flashlight."

The two started out toward the back of the garage, trying to keep out of sight rather than startle what or who was hiding. Suddenly, a man started running toward the neighbor's house, jumping over low shrubs, headed for the neighbor's back porch . As he reached the porch, he knocked over a flower planter which crashed on the cement.

"Hey, you!" yelled Tom Tucker, the owner of the property. "Stand still; I'm coming out." Alex was sprawled on the cement driveway, covered in potting soil and flowers. Josh and Jed were right next to him, trying to help him to his feet.

Alex, however, wasn't having anything to do with this plan. He tried to get away from his sons but they held firm.

"Let me go! Can't you see he's trying to kill me? He's been following me every night with his gun. I saw it! I saw it!"

Tom just shook his head. "I knew Alex had been doing some kind of skullduggery out there every night. But why would he think I was going to kill him?"

The sons were at a loss for words. They each took one of Alex's arms and started to lead him home.

"No, no," he cried, obviously very frightened. "I know what he's trying to do. He's going to make you think he's a friend, but he really hates me!"

Enough. You get the picture. It seems that there had been several such incidents over the preceding three months, but they happened during the hours when the sons were out of the house and their Mom was getting some well-deserved sleep. Alex was sneaking out the back door, trying to escape the demons he saw and heard... the evil men (including Tom) who were trying to kill him. Other neighbors had called the police on two occasions but they never found anyone when they made their routine pass through the area.

This case is a true one. It's been pretty well camouflaged, but it is true. The person in question had been experiencing dreadful, scary hallucinations which repeated night after night. Finally placed in a long term care facility, medications had to be used on a regular basis to allow both the victim and other residents to have a more serene life.

Alex died less than a year after the incident just described.

I think it's time for another intermission. I'm getting thirsty and my dear husband has put on a pot of coffee.

How do I know? Almond Amaretto is wafting upwards!

GETTING BACK TO "OLD TIMERS" DISEASE

G etting back to that gentleman at the Grange
meeting... you thought I'd forgotten, didn't you!
Well, this wasn't the first time I had heard "Alzheimer,"
spoken with a bit of guttural 't ' as a substitute for 'zhe,'
by many people, regardless of age.

I suppose it makes sense. It's mostly old timers that
get it. But that isn't entirely true in the 21st century. (I
wonder if Buck Rogers ever had dementia. Oh. He was
in the 25th century. Sorry.)

Mr. Dzierkewicz was really correct. His name, by
the way, is a combination of the various consonants and
syllables of many of the Polish names whose families
settled in beautiful Western Massachusetts and still
farm here today, No actual person.

The old 'general suspected cases' list (that's not the
real name statisticians use, but it is easier to pronounce,
used to say 5% under 65. 65-70 10%; 70-75 15%; 75-80
20%; 80-85 25% to 30%. By 85, nearly 50%. As you
can see, it is truly an "old timers" disease.

I learned recently that if there is a genetic component in your family history, if you make it to 70 or 75, there is little chance that the genetic type will kick in. That may not be too helpful to those of you who are breathing a breath of relief, only to be told that your chances of 'catching' Alzheimer's is up to 25%+ by 75.

So, yes, the majority of people who have this type of dementia are usually in the late end of middle age or the early side of old age. Since we not believe that the cohort known as the "very old" are usually 85 years + you can see that we have to juggle statistics as each decade passes.

Think about it. If you are in your 70s now, you are probably very active, either still working… because you love your work, or you need money to live…and often you may be spending more time in volunteer work than you ever did while "punching the time clock."

Now think back to when you were in grammar school. Do you remember your grand parents? They were old, weren't they? Very old? Like maybe in their 50s? You may have even had great grand parents, if you were lucky. Now *that* is really old.

I think of the birth notices that are printed each day in our local paper. (That tells you that I live in a really old fashioned place, doesn't it?) As I glance through the names, it is NOT the parent's names I look for. It's the grand parents and greats. I know that I have a class reunion coming up next year. #60. As I see the names, I realize that a great many of the great grands are classmates. These are the same people who live in Florida or some other southern locale in the winter. I happen to believe that if you are a true New Englander, winter is part and parcel of your blood line. But, once again, I digress.

These 'snow birds' as they are called, spend their days at the golf course, playing tennis, bridge, sailing, or... if they are real New Englanders, skiing, cross country most likely, swimming at the Y, or maybe working out. Mall walking is very popular around here. Keeps you away from the icy streets and roads. The point being that grand parents today are active, alert, interested in community as well as family. If you were to look at a picture of your great grand parents at the time you thought they were exceedingly old, and then picked up a digital photo of people at that age today, you would quickly realize that "these aren't your mother's old people!"

When I hear that someone's mother or father-in-law has withdrawn from activities they previously enjoyed, or that they have a kind of blankness in their conversation and attentiveness, I begin to think that this person, perhaps, needs to be watched. I have seen too many instances in which that person has 'given up' the chore of trying to keep it all a secret. It's like the questions which came following the letter from President Ronald Reagan announcing to the world that he had Alzheimer's. I was actively working at that time and several of my colleagues and I were talking of his announcement. Each person at the gathering had the same idea: how long has this been going on? Looking back at various periods some five years previous to his announcement, there were clues, if you knew what to be looking for. This may not have been true, but those of us who worked nearly 24/7 with families in which dementia ruled most of their lives, could see the warning signs.

And because of that, and because there are still a huge percentage of individuals who think that dementia is just part of the aging process, "old timers" "Alzheimers" is pooh-poohed. It's supposed to be part of being old. Forget about it. As the old doc told one man, "She's got Alzheimer's (this diagnosis done without any testing at all) so just take her home and care of her. We can't do anything about it."

This probably would be an acceptable scenario were it 1940. Back then, the doctor would have used the words, "hardening of the arteries" or "organic brain syndrome."

I am reminded of a meeting I attended in 1985 (I believe that was the year) at the Brattleboro Retreat in Vermont. This was an all day seminar by a well known physician, professor, researcher, all rolled into one. His name was Barry Reisberg and he was one of an early group of individuals who could see that dementia was a lot more than just part of growing old, as many believed. His presentation that day included a broad scope of topics but one thing he said has remained in my mind. He spoke of the absence of any information on dementia in the long list of ailments which a young physician might see. He told us of his own days in medical school and beyond. He pointed out that in a 2,000 page textbook on *Neurology*, Alzheimer's disease was given approximately one paragraph. That was in 1969, according to the good doctor. In 1984, times had changed! There were two *pages* in the similar size text.

That was the situation only about twenty-two years ago. Can you imagine?

You can see why so many people, including health professionals, don't seem too upset when a loved one is diagnosed with dementia, particularly of the Alzheimer type. If the physician in question had been in medical school when the tidal wave of information spewed out to the world, he/she might well have heard in passing that a lot of people were getting Alzheimer's. The usual response might be "what?"

Dr. Reisberg continues his work. His Global Deterioration Scale is used world-wide to determine the staging of the impaired person. Not satisfied with the usual 'early – mid – late' stage diagnoses, his seven steps give a more precise picture of what will be happening to the person so diagnosed. It has been of great assistance to the thousands, probably millions, now working in the field of dementia.

Not resting on his laurels, he has since described the losses in Alzheimer's as following the precise order in which these capabilities are mastered in the infant and child. We can, therefore, look to the incapacitated elder with Alzheimer's to lose the ability to walk before losing the ability to speak. I'll talk about his term, "retrogenesis" in another chapter.

The word to all those at the Grange meetings, the Senior Centers, the Rotarians, Kiwanians and assorted animal groups of Lions, Elks, Moose, etc. who may be hearing for the first time the true facts on dementia will be benefiting from the work of researchers like Reisberg, Roses, Selkoe, Albert, Tanzi, Small, and Whitehouse:.

Alzheimer's Disease is NOT part of the aging process!

My list of researchers is compiled of just those who came to mind without looking at a text. I have over fifty volumes in my own personal library and admit to having a fetish for treatises on all types of dementia. You will find in my alphabetized list of cases that I've run into some truly rare causes of dementia.

The other problem which has been nagging those of us who consider dementia their life work is the difference between dementia and Alzheimer's. I can't tell you how many times I have overheard a family member say, "Thank God he doesn't have Alzheimer's! The doctor said it's just dementia."

That makes as much sense as "The report said she has carcinoma of the colon. We are so happy it's not cancer."

Bad enough we have to correct those kind-hearted folk who insist that Alzheimer's is that terrible disease and dementia is just forgetting where you left your glasses. If that were true, then I must have been demented for some 70 years or more, since I had my first spectacles at the tender age of six. I presently have computer glasses which are an in between range; I have three pair of drugstore reading glasses which I may or may not need, depending on the size of the type. I have bifocals which I really don't need but since they change as soon as they are hit by sunlight, they are good to have around. And last, I have my regular sunglasses.

(Whether you have had cataracts removed or not, wear some good sunglasses year round.)

Please note that these glasses have not caused dementia; however, I continue to forget where I last saw which pair. Having a patient husband is very helpful. As to the actual problem, here's my way of looking at the situation.

DEMENTIA

A group of symptoms which include memory loss, difficulties with numbers, problems with language: speaking, understanding including reading and writing, changes in personality and behavior.

NOT A PART OF NORMAL AGING

Think of the term Dementia as a big umbrella of symptoms. There are a number of causes of dementia, so picture them as ribbons attached to the inside ribs of the umbrella. Considering how many causes there are, maybe we should be picturing a tarp big enough to cover Fenway Park!

Most experts agree that Alzheimer's disease is the primary cause of dementia. That old time doc that mentioned 'hardening of the arteries' might have been referring to "Vascular Dementia" or "Multi-Infarct Dementia." We know that there is a dementia caused by problems in the arterial system… that is one reason why you hear so much about your cholesterol levels and a relationship to dementia. If you have lots of plaque floating around, it might just clog up a necessary connection of blood to a part of your brain. Not good.

To make it even worse, there is a Combo: Alzheimer's and Vascular in one person. You get the worst of both diseases. Added to those three types, recent years have identified another charming player: Lewy Body Dementia. This one is a mixed bag of the symptoms of both Alzheimer's and Parkinson's Disease. Just something to muddy up the diagnostic picture.

If it wasn't enough to have Lewy Bodies causing problems (a more complete description in the Alphabetic Stories), we also have Frontotemporal Dementias or Frontal Lobe Dementias, that being the front of your head... like forehead? ...and a whole kit and caboodle of players here: Pick's is the one most heard about in the general public but there are a string of weird-sounding names that also fit in here.

Let's not forget the ever popular Mad Cow Disease. Actually, the correct name for that is Creutzfeldt-Jacob v (for variant). But the main category of Creutzfeldt-Jacob Disease may occur cowless. It's a terrible disease caused by a *PRION* which is smaller that a virus. If you remember by earlier description of the size differences between bacteria and virus, you can understand that something smaller than a virus is getting pretty close to infinitesimal. But, boy, can it cause trouble!

After that menu of badies, we should point out to some two hundred plus others to think about. But we're not going to do that. It would take a great deal of explaining and, as good environmentalist, I don't want to kill too many trees.

Let's finish off this little koffee klatch by saying, you can get a multitude of information by checking with your local chapter of the Alzheimer's Association.

I believe you'll find them in the phone book. If not, go on line to *www.alz.org.*

THE ALPHABET SOUP PEOPLE

D uring the past many years when I was speaking to a group or writing one of my columns, I insisted on breaking with the tradition of naming people by calling them "Adam #1 J" or "Shirley #2 S" to allow for privacy issues. I always thought it was dumb to use the person's first name and some notation that they were the first or second (or more) in the data base with the same name or initials. Besides, it takes too long to even explain the system!

My method is simpler. People are named with the first letter of the alphabet for a fictitious first name and the second letter of the alphabet for their second name. You saw this in the "Alice... Carla... Eliza" story. So if I start the following segment of this book with full first and last names, you will realize that the names I have chosen are simply that: names out of my active imagination. In many cases, if the particular case in question might still be recognizable (by whom, I can't imagine), then we change their sex, make them older or younger, and probably move them to another part of the country. It's kind of like the game of chess. You get to move people around and play the master of this particular universe. But before we continue with our story, here are a few words from our sponsor. **M E**

I watched a television show on CBS this evening. (I'm a night writer. That's not the same as a sky writer. Or a night walker.) In this 'police drama' a female officer enters an interrogation room with another woman, the daughter-in-law of an older woman who was found dead in a fire. The conversation, brief though it is, tells a story.

"So, did your mother have Alzheimer's?" asked the police officer. "No," replies the other woman, "She had senile dementia." I am ready to contact CBS tomorrow! Is it too much of a task to get the right words? Really, now!

Here we go, folks. It's show time!

The Alphabet People

A B   Arthur Banratty Alzheimer's? Senility?
C D   Claire Dunwoody Down related Alzheimer's
E F   Edwin Flynt Early Onset Alzheimer's
G H   Grace Hanrihan Combined form Alzheimer's
I J   Isaac Jacobson Late Onset (Sporadic)
       Alzheimer's
K L   Ken Ludwig Amyotrophic Lateral Sclerosis
M N   Mendal Neuberg Binswanger's Disease
O P   Ophelia Plantar Creutzfeldt-Jacob Disease
Q R   Quinn Rogers Frontotemporal Dementia
S T   Steve Tomaski Huntington's Disease
U V   Una Vasquez Klüver-Bucy Syndrome
W Y   Walt Yankowski Lewy Body Dementia

The Reversed Alphabet People

B A   Betty Android Lupus: Neurologic Sequelae

109

D C   Donald Chapin Mitochondrial Myopathies

F E   Fred Elgar Vascular/Multi-Infarct Dementia

H G   Harriet Grover Multiple Sclerosis

J I   Jake Interman Normal Pressure Hydrocephalus

L K   Lena Kowalski Parkinson's Disease

N M   Naomi Ming Pick's Disease

P O   Pedro Ortez Progressive Suprenuclear Palsy

R Q   Rebecca Quinlan Stroke

T S   Ted Sanford Transient Ischemic Attack (TIA)

V U   Venita Usher Transmissible Spongiform Encephalopathies

Y W   Yancy Waters Wernicke-Korsakoff Syndrome

A B Arthur Banratty—Alzheimer's? Or Senility'?

Arthur's wife, Mattilda, insisted her 70 year old husband was "senile" and she wouldn't hear otherwise. She was not a feisty woman. She was NASTY and the social worker who had joined me in this home visit agreed with me totally as we spoke after driving away from the house.

This couple lived some distance from our home office. In fact they were in a very small town in the center of the State. We had received the referral from another Area Agency on Aging closer to the Banratty home.

Now, it seems that Tildy, as she liked to be called, had her own way of looking at things. Arthur was a retired postal clerk who was happy to stay at home and put his feet up. She wanted him to go on trips with her. ALL the time.

Arthur also liked to spend a great deal of his time reading. Tildy didn't read. I don't mean to infer that she was illiterate, although she proudly admitted she hadn't read anything but the local newspaper since she finished high school, some 50+ years ago. (She also admitted that she only read the obituaries in the paper.)

Tildy said Arthur must be senile because he didn't remember anything she told him. He must be senile because it took him so long to do anything. He didn't shower every day. He didn't wear a shirt and tie. He didn't talk with her friends. He was totally distracted.

She reported that when she told him yesterday that there was going to be a pot luck supper at church today, he said, "What Church?"

Sarah and I spoke privately with Arthur. We had asked if Tildy would mind if we did our own assessment of her husband and she smiled broadly saying, "Oh, that's fine. He can't keep any secrets from me anyhow."

My colleague started asking a few simple questions about his day to day life. All we got in response was Tildy's answers from the next room! You see the problem.

This episode happened nearly ten years ago. I saw the two of them a few weeks back and had to chuckle. Tildy was in a wheelchair, bland affect, being pushed down the grocery store aisles by Arthur.

Alzheimer's is in the picture, but it isn't Arthur. He has stuck it out all these years, playing the role of Casper Milquetoast, a comic character none of you remember, unless you were born before World War II.

Arthur used to say "Yes, dear," very often. No more. He goes about his business and doesn't have to respond to Tildy's every word.

Arthur's memory was perfectly fine, as was his hearing. He just tuned out. His belief was that he had worked over 40 years when he retired and had no intention of "spinning my wheels to keep her happy." He dressed as he pleased. He didn't shower every day because his doctor told him he didn't need to... and shouldn't dry out his skin. He read the books he had always wanted to read and became almost a daily fixture at the Public Library.

So this was an easy one. A case of the hen-pecked husband trying to keep himself protected against a life he chose not to lead.

Marriage counseling, perhaps.

Alzheimer's? NO!

CD Claire Dunwoody—Down related Alzheimers

Claire lives at home with her aging parents. Now 45, she has been working at the local supermarket for a number of years through a community placement program. The family was called in to talk with the manager when other workers noticed she was no longer able to follow directions and was becoming unable to remember what the clerks had told her to do.

Down syndrome is a known risk factor for dementia, up there with aging and other genetic related forms. Individuals with chromosome 21 trisomy, or Down's syndrome, express the APP gene at 150 percent of normal throughout their life and essentially all develop neuropatholigical lesions of Alzheimer's disease by the age of 40, including both amyloid plaques and neurofibrillary tangles.

Some studies indicate that nearly 100% of Down patients eventually will show the signs and symptoms of dementia by age 50. In Down related dementia, the time between diagnosis and death is about half the normal time attributed to sporadic Alzheimer's and many will die within five years.

Recognizing that Claire would not be able to continue her work placement at the supermarket, her parents met with the social worker assigned to their daughter. They knew that as their 78th and 79th birthdays were approaching, a plan needed to be formulated to care for Claire after their death. The planning had to be done now.

Fortunately, the community in which Claire lived had a very active association combined of professionals in the field as well as family members who were dedicated to maintaining programs for their children, no matter the age.

The new "House and Home" building which had been built with a grant from the State and maintained through funds from the Department of Mental Retardation (a title the families were attempting to have changed) would be open in about six weeks. Claire had visited there with other members of the older group of impaired individuals and had come home to her parents raving about this great place! Knowing her reaction, the parents started the process of arranging for her to be one of those lucky people who would be moving to "our own house" as Claire said.

Things don't always work this way. In fact, in too many cases, this kind of placement would probably take many years on a waiting list. Older parents of offspring with a developmental disorder need to look into what is available in their own community, knowing in their heart that the time will come when such a change will become a necessity.

Planning ahead is always wise; not many people ever really do it. We all tend to put off until tomorrow and too often, tomorrow surprises us by arriving too soon.

Many organizations working with this group of adults have information available to guardians and parents. Some offer training programs or a series of teaching events so that those caring for an impaired person are up to date on current laws in their area. We have fifty States and I doubt that any have the same laws in place.

In Claire's case, she moved into "House and Home" and has thrived in that type of care situation. She continues to exhibit signs of dementia and the staff at this program have been trained to realize that the protocol used in dealing with the developmentally disabled, a protocol which relies heavily on memory, is no longer applicable. Hard as it is to change the direction of the mind of a disabled person, it is often much harder to change the mind set of a professional!

People with retardation, even though their entire life has had them pigeon-holed as 'developmentally disabled', must now be cared for as a person whose brain has been effected in another manner: dementia is now their primary diagnosis.

Claire is doing well, when last I spoke with the parents. It's nice to see a story with a happy ending. It doesn't happen often enough.

EF Edwin Flynt — Early Onset Alzheimers

Edwin held a prominent position in the community. He was president of one of the local banks and chaired many civic organizations. He and his wife were parents of three adult children, all living away from home.

One day, a close friend and colleague who held a similar position in another financial institution, called Ed's wife, asking if they could meet to talk. She was a bit taken aback by his request and pressed him as to why they couldn't get together at her home when Ed was available. He spoke calmly in response, telling her that it involved Edwin and that it would be better if she could meet him somewhere, anywhere but at her house.

You can just imagine all the things that went through her mind. When Ed came home that evening, she chose not to mention the phone call. She did, however, take a good look at her husband, listened to his usual banter of bits and pieces of work and local gossip, and still could not see that there was any problem.

The following morning, she drove to a coffee shop on the edge of Town. Their good friend was waiting for her and they took seats on benches opposite each other. "What is it," she said. "Why do we have to meet like this?"

"This is not easy to say and you probably won't believe what I'm going to tell you. Ed can no longer continue to work. He has lost the ability to understand numbers."

"That's impossible. He has an M.B.A. from the University of Pennsylvania. You mean to tell me that this man who has spent the last 25 years of his life working in finance *can't understand numbers???*" You're out of your mind! How dare you insinuate that Ed can't do his job. That's pure nonsense!"

He waited while she processed what she had heard, still denying that such a thing could happen to Edwin. As the anger turned to anxiety and tears, he moved to her side of the table and held her hand, patting her shoulder as she tried to control her emotions.

As a result of this incident, Ed's wife spoke with the other officers at Ed's bank by phone. She told him of what she had just learned and asked their opinion on the situation. They all agreed that he had certainly lost his usual flair; they had   noticed that he managed to have someone else take over in a situation in which he didn't feel comfortable. She asked that they not mention to Ed that she had called and also requested that they not confront Ed about the problem until she had a chance to speak with their physician. They agreed but also urged her to tell Edwin of what they all had noticed… the sooner the better.

She called their doctor immediately and asked to speak with him personally on a grave matter. He called her back within ten minutes. He hadn't seen Ed for nearly a year. In fact, it was time for his physical. No, he told her, he was not aware of any problem with Ed's brain, but things can change, you know.

Ed came home that evening, totally unaware that he had become the center of a maelstrom which would eventually change his life completely.

The next day, after undergoing a thorough physical examination, including blood work, an ECG, and scheduling of a colonoscopy, his doctor brought him into his private office and told him he thought he might be having some kind of memory problem.

"Now, don't worry, Ed. It's probably nothing. You seem to be quite healthy. Are you feeling down or anxious about anything?" the doctor asked.

Edwin looked at his old friend, saying, "You know something, don't you. You know that I'm having a problem at work. I don't know why. I don't know what it is, but numbers are acting strangely. No. That doesn't make sense, does it?"

"I'd like you to see a special kind of doctor. No, not a psychiatrist. But the name is almost hard to pronounce: he's a neuropsychologist. You'll do some routine tests like those we used to do with putting pieces of a puzzle together, doing some naming of objects... nothing you have to worry about. I'll set the testing up for the first part of next week. In the meantime, just go home, take a couple of vacation days and relax. We'll get this straightened out."

When the testing was complete, Edwin was diagnosed with early onset Alzheimer's. He was 49 years old.

Early onset Alzheimer's is a rare form of dementia that strikes people younger than age 65. Though no clear scientific reason for this age break currently exists, it has been adopted by convention and consensus. The manifestation of early onset is similar to those of the disease in older adults. Since we don't normally expect to see someone in the 40s or 50s having dementia, problems often emerge at work and in the home and are wrongly mistaken as lack of motivation, alcoholism or a psychiatric problem. These people may lose relationships or be fired, losing their medical benefits. Early diagnostic testing is imperative.

Early onset forms seem more likely to have an autosomal dominant pattern of genetic transmission. All genes currently known to cause Alzheimers are of early onset form. Obviously, there are huge problems connected with this type of dementia. How does the family survive financially? How do you cope with younger children? What sources are available for day care?

Edwin has been in a nursing home for five years, at this writing. The end is near. Those with early onset often have a much shorter life span.

His family is doing well. His youngest child, a son, completed college during the time his dad was in the nursing home and has returned home to work in the Town and be with his mother during this difficult... no, dreadful, time.

GH Grace Hanrihan —Combined form
Alzheimers

Grace was a retired school teacher (no relation to our friend Alice who is Eliza's Mom) who enjoyed traveling with others who were also widows or former teachers.

She was also the life of the party! Her sense of humor had worked well while still teaching and many years later, it remained a part of her personality.

She was 80 when her family first noticed a problem. For her birthday, her nieces took her to lunch at a well known restaurant down near the Connecticut line. One of her gifts was a tulip plant in full bloom. It was artificial, but certainly looked just like a true flower.

She tried to pour the water in her glass into the potted plant. Later, she made quite a scene by calling out in a loud voice, "Look at that silly blouse" while pointing at a woman seated nearby.

This was not the Grace we had all come to know and love. The nieces tried to calm the atmosphere. The elder of the three women went to the next table and quietly explained that their aunt was having mental difficulties and she did not really mean what she had said. She apologized profusely and returned to her seat. The middle niece caught the eye of the waiter and asked for the check. The youngest woman went to the check room to pick up their coats. I think they were hoping that either a power outage would occur so that they could sneak out, or that some other diner would have a baby on the spot! Anything to draw attention away from Grace and her 'new' personality.

What to do? I don't mean about the ruined meal. What to do about Grace's fall from 'grace'. The only close relative was a step-son who lived in central Massachusetts... and since he was not a blood relative, the nieces didn't know if he would be of help or not. Whatever was to be done, it seemed that having Grace seen by her physician would be the first step. But how to get her there?

Grace lived in an apartment building near the center of Town. There were several other teachers living in that building and they all would get together every morning at 10:00 for coffee and talk. One woman, in particular, was the self-appointed head of the group. That might be because she was in her late 80s and decided that age has its own rules.

The elder niece, we'll call her Geraldine, called the head teacher and asked if she had noted any changes in Grace over the past few months.

"Well, now, I wondered when someone would mention her problem. She's straight off to the Loony bin!" she replied. "We've known for months now that she can't remember a thing, sometimes dresses funny and had a chip on her shoulder... or not... depending on which day of the week it is."

Geraldine knew why this particular woman was the self-named head of the group. Age had nothing to do with it. She was just a born leader and didn't put up with any nonsense from anyone. Just the person to get behind her plan to get Grace to the doctor.

"We have noticed that she's not herself; in fact, I have an appointment set up for this afternoon with her doctor, but I wonder if I'm going to have a hard time getting her to go?" said Geraldine. "Do you have any thoughts?"

"Of course I do! Why don't we just stop over at her apartment and I can tell her that she's been acting funny and we think she should see her doctor and find out what's wrong with her."

Geraldine was not accustomed to speaking with someone who was so certain in her mind that getting Grace to the doctor was like getting up in the morning. You just DO it. The plan was set and both women descended on Grace at 2:00 p.m.

"Come on, Grace. We're driving you to an appointment with your doctor. Get your things together." Geraldine was speechless, yet was able to tell her aunt that she did, in fact, have an appointment and that her friend wanted to go along for the drive. Ah, yes. The methods of communication some people use... and seem to get away with.

The trip to the doctor's office was quiet. It seemed as though everyone had their own thoughts but decided against speaking. When they arrived, Geraldine went to the reception desk and said that Grace was ready for her appointment and that she would like to speak with the doctor after the examination because of behavioral problems which had been noted by her friends.

Grace was on good behavior that day. She happened to like her doctor, a man she had known some thirty years. Off she went to the examining room. A nurse came out about ten minutes later to tell her that Grace wanted her to join her in the room.

Geraldine caught the doctor's eye as she came in and there was a very slight nod to let her know that he was aware of the problems even without speaking to the niece.

The outcome of this visit was that Grace now knew that she probably had some memory problems and that she would need to be seen by a few other people who would help her plan for some help in her home. Of course Grace didn't believe that she needed anyone or anything.

Returning Grace to her apartment, Geraldine decided to take a look around. She asked if Grace would like a cold drink (a ploy to get into the refrigerator) and with a quick glance, she saw baking soda, a dried up piece of cheese, a small container of unknown origin and a very decayed, green orange. You get the picture.

After about half an hour, Geraldine was more than ready to start contacting agencies, relatives, and a lawyer. This was going to be another of those cases.

There were services put in place; a woman would do grocery shopping for Grace and Meals on Wheels was contacted to provide a noon meal five days a week. The teachers in the building volunteered to cover the weekends for at least two meals. There was to be a homemaker to come in three times a week to do dishes, laundry, and some cleaning. This was to be paid for though Grace's own funds, and the actual bookkeeping was to be taken care of by the step-son. He volunteered to come up every weekend to check on Grace and to take care of removing her car.

The holiday season was approaching. Winter in New England can be brutal, even to New Englanders. Although it hadn't snowed in early December, the eldest niece had a phone call from the U.S. Postal Service. It seems that one of the clerks had looked out the window and saw Grace walking down the street. She had on a pair of soft bedroom slippers, a slip as an undergarment and a light weight jacket, probably to a summer outfit. He knew that her apartment was in the building around the corner from the Post Office and sent one of the women clerks out to lead Grace back home. By calling the niece, he let her know that someone should be contacted to stay with her immediately. The temperature was 20°. There are benefits to living in a small Town.

Not long after that event, a guardian was appointed by the Court and Grace entered a long term care facility in the same Town.

Did you think this was the end of the Grace story? No, way! She hadn't been there a week when someone in the building warned staff that Grace had decided to go home. Out the front door, dressed to the nines, hat and purse with her, she had been missed... or been mistaken for a visitor.

The staff (administration, that is) took off in their car, feeling that she was probably headed for the main road into the Town. When the sound of brakes and horns being blown reached them, they knew they had found Grace. She was walking up the down ramp of Route 91.

Go forward about three years. By this time, Grace was pretty much incommunicado. She had her own language which, to most, sounded like gibberish. She had a small color TV in her room and watched Sesame Street every morning, chattering to her animals and dolls as though she were still teaching.

On a more anxiety producing occasion (it was staff that was anxious), Grace came out of her room, pocketbook in hand, and walked over to another resident who was quietly seated, watching the passing parade. He was an elderly gentleman who certainly didn't deserve to be pummeled over the head by this feisty woman with her pocketbook.

Some of you may remember a TV show known as "Laugh In" in 1968 ... you will recognize the scenario: Ruth Buzzi comes over to Arte Johnson, the Little Old Man, who is sitting on a park bench. Buzzi starts hitting him over the head while he mumbles some response.

This was a frequent event and the staff was at the end of their proverbial rope, trying to figure out the source of the problem. Finally they called Niece #1.

After she arrived at the home, listened to the story, then asked to be shown the poor man in question, she started laughing. Have you ever tried to laugh when there are people all around and no one else gets the joke?

It seems that the pummeled person was the "spitting image" of the man who used to take Grace's husband to a certain bar every day after work. Grace always said that if she ever got her hands on him, he'd have something to think about!

Well, Grace wasn't thinking, the man wasn't thinking, and if he were, he would say that he wished he didn't look anything like the pal of this mad woman's former husband!

This time it IS the end. Grace died in the same nursing home nine years later.

I J Isaac Jacobson—Late Onset (Sporadic) Alzheimer's

Isaac lived most of his life in the Boston area. His law practice kept him very busy and his partners became concerned when he showed up for trial one day, totally unprepared. Beautifully dressed, correct posture, handling himself as he had for decades, the Judge noted his lapse in formality in response to being questioned.

Although only 68, looking ten years younger, Isaac could not answer a simple question. A partner in the firm who was sitting first chair, called for a recess. He spoke with the Judge and requested a postponement since Isaac was going immediately to Mass. General (better known in the world as Massachusetts General Hospital). There, Isaac was admitted for observation and testing.

While there, the family was called together. Isaac's wife had been keeping Isaac's condition from the family and from his law partners, believing that he just needed some time off... a nice vacation, maybe. (Perhaps a trip down the Nile? Remember: Denial is more than a river in Egypt.)

Isaac closed out his business relationships and he and his wife moved to western Massachusetts where they have now lived (with a high degree of help) in a small town in the south of the Connecticut River Valley. Now in the late stages of Alzheimer's, his placement in a special dementia facility will be very soon.

Anyone who has cared for an Alzheimer patient is aware that the disease is insidious. Many times the impaired person can cover up their losses. Coupled with a degree of denial on the part of the care giver, it usually takes some incident to bring everyone to a realization of the victim's condition.

Following the Global Deterioration Scale which has been mentioned before, the symptoms which become manifest in Stage 5 of Dr. Reisberg's instrument, are those which are most prominent when the word becomes: SOMETHING HAS TO BE DONE! We often find that the more intelligent the person, the less others will be able to recognize the dementia. There have been those with a score of 25 (out of 30) on the Mini-Mental Status Exam (MMSE) who were actually in mid-stage Alzheimer's. While 68 is on the young side for developing AD, it can happen. 79 – 85 would be more the norm, while 70 – 79 would be the earlier stage of the disease. But, every person is different. There are no cookie cutters here.

When I last spoke with Isaac's wife, she told me that they were getting along quite well. I thought of Nancy Reagan, who certainly could have twenty-four hour help while caring for the late President. With all the available assistance, she showed the stress of caring when she appeared on various television broadcasts. This is a hard, hard disease with which caregivers are faced. It can be rationalized that "I can take care of my loved one with help from others." Having the means to do it and having the fortitude to watch a person disintegrate before your eyes is not as easy as it seems.

As I was writing this chapter, I heard that his wife had moved from the home they owned into an assisted living residence. While I did not pry as to the reason for the move, I presume Isaac has moved also, and probably to the specialized unit outside the Town.

K L Ken Ludwig—Amyotrophic Lateral Sclerosis

I could have named him Lou Gehrig and you would automatically know the story. Ken was a car salesman. Married, with two grown children, he was 52 when he started having symptoms: he tripped while going up into the bleachers at the hockey rink.

Then, he had difficulty walking any distance. He used to love golf, but it became impossible to play, even with a cart. His doctor told him he was clumsy and suggested that he go to the gym and build up his muscles.

One morning, he couldn't get out of bed. When his wife tried to help him, he told her there was nothing wrong... he was just extremely tired. Staying at home, he had to give up his job. Finally, his daughter insisted that he be tested at Baystate Medical Center in Springfield. There, they quickly diagnosed ALS and put him on the new medication Riluzole® which helps delay the symptoms of ALS.

Once again, we had a fairly young man whose disease uprooted his family. His wife had to go to work and the two adult children changed their plans. They offered to stay with him whenever his wife was away from the house.

Many friends from the days when Ken coached hockey came to his aid. He was able to remain at home until the paralysis had taken over most of his body and his brain became involved in the progression of the disease.

Amyotrophic Lateral Sclerosis (ALS) or "Lou Gehrig's disease" is a progressive, fatal neurological disease affecting about 20,000 in the USA with 5,000 new cases each year. (ALS us usually fatal within five years of diagnosis.)

Known as a motor neuron disease, ALS occurs when specific nerve cells (which control voluntary movement) in the brain and spinal cord gradually degenerate. This loss causes muscle to weaken and waste away, leading to paralysis. Symptoms may include tripping and falling, loss of motor control in hands and arms, difficulty speaking, swallowing and breathing, persistent fatigue and twitching and cramping of muscles.

Men are about one and a half times more likely to have the disease as are women. In some cases, dementia results when certain brain sections become involved. This is more likely in very late stages but does involve memory losses.

I have included this particular story because I watched a colleague deal with this disorder and watched his brave family care for him in his home until his death. They deserve great praise for what they believe to be "what we should do… we love him… we care for him."

M N Mendal Neuberg—Binswanger's Disease

Mendal is one of my favorite people. I first met him about ten years ago at the symphony. His wife was on the board and was my sister's friend.

What a delight! I used to kid him about taking energy pill for breakfast. He was active in his work, in the community and a true "gym rat" in the "Cardiac Club" at the Y.

He had a mild "cardiac event' as he called it, about a dozen years ago and he was bound that he would still be playing golf at age 90. He was only 65 at the time.

I hadn't seen him for several years and wondered what had happened in his life. My sister filled me in.

Mendal had what appeared to be a small stroke. He became clumsy, slow in speech, had difficulty walking and (to his dismay) became incontinent. It wasn't related to prostate surgery. What could it be?

He decided to go to the University of Massachusetts Medical Center in Worcester for a neurologic workup. They told him it was Binswanger's disease, which is supposedly rare, although you hear more and more of people being diagnosed. Because of his urinary problems and inability to 'be himself' as he said, he had become quite reclusive and didn't want to go out in public. His wife was in the process of placing him in a long term care facility.

Binswangers is referred to as a subcortical dementia, characterized by cerebrovascular lesions in the deep white matter of the brain, loss of memory and cognition, mood changes and often signs of abnorma blood vessels in the neck as well as disease of the heart valves. There is often incontinence, difficulty walking, clumsiness, slowness of conduct, lack of facial expression and speech difficulties. There is no specific course of this slowly progressive condition and death usually occurs less than ten years after diagnosis.

Although this is the usual description of the presentation and course of Binswangers, the jury seems to be out. I know that many sources report that Binswangers is a rare type of vascular dementia, more and more clinicians are pointing to an increased number of well diagnosed cases during the past five years of the 21st century. Is it not rare? Is it being misdiagnosed? Or are these just sporadic anecdotal reports? Perhaps the advances in imagery, allowing for more definitive differential diagnoses have brought Binswangers to the forefront. Keep watching. We may learn more.

O P Ophelia Plantar—Creutzfeldt-Jacob Disease

If another Grant Wood would like to paint an American Gothic picture, pitchfork and all, then Ophella would have made a perfect model. She was a spinster lady living outside the tiny village of Buckland,   in the hills of Franklin County. She kept sheep and loved gardening and spinning that special wool from her darlings. As long as you spoke kindly about animals, you could be a friend.

She had a niece who lived in eastern Massachusetts but always visited, particularly on holidays. Thanksgiving at Ophelia's brought together many of the locals as well as Susan, the niece.

Shortly before Labor Day about five years ago, Susan had a call from one of the old timers in Buckland. Something was wrong with Ophelia. She was unable to walk out to the barn without falling, didn't seem to know the man who delivered the mail and wouldn't talk with anyone.

Susan hightailed it to Buckland. She was not welcomed by her aunt. Ophelia wouldn't open the door. What to do? How to get help? Susan put a call into her aunt's doctor who called for an ambulance and assistance from the local police. It was not a pretty scene.

After gaining entrance, they found Ophelia on the floor, unable to get up, appearing frightened of everyone. She was transported to the local hospital where she was put in quarantine until some diagnosis was made. Here's what caused this:

Creutzfeldt-Jacob disease is a rare, degenerative, invariably fatal brain disorder. Onset usually occurs at about age 60. There are three categories: sporadic, hereditary and acquired. There is no diagnostic test. Ruling out encephalitis or meningitis (both occur in the brain) is the usual treatment.

Opiate drugs are used to help relieve the pain of jerking muscles. 90% die within a year. Patients have failing memory, behavioral changes, lack of coordination and mental deterioration. There is pronounced involuntary movements, blindness, weakness and coma.

While not usually communicable, Emery University Hospital in Georgia had to contact some 500 patients who might have been exposed to CJD by surgical instruments infected with CJD. The prion element which causes this disease is not touched by usual types of sterilization. You may remember when I spoke of a prion earlier in this book.

Creutzfeldt-Jacob: Think Mad Cow Disease.

When speaking of "Mad Cow" we should point out that the correct term is bovine spongiform encephalopathy. That seen in humans is usually CJDv meaning it is a variant of Creutzfeldt-Jacob. We may see these terms mixed as scientists look to the connections between animal and human. The recent news on Avian Flu, also known as Asian Avian Flu, is that there are no documented cases of the animal (or fowl) type being transferred to humans. As I write in 2006, we are becoming more and more aware of virus diseases and probably those caused by prions as well.

Mad Cow Disease has been given a dual role in our culture. While it is a distinctive and dangerous disease, at the same time, it has become fodder for the late night comedians and even cartoonists.

Remember my story of Ophelia. Then watch what the media produces.

Q R Quinn Rogers—Frontotemporal Dementia

The Honorable Quinn Rogers was the Presiding Justice of the Probate and Family Court in Rockland County. In his early 60s, his colleagues on the bench became concerned when he exhibited a drastic personality change, including suspiciousness, nearing paranoia. He accused lawyers before him of trying to trick him and accused his Clerk of trying to put something in his coffee.

Fortunately, the Probate Court often deals with individuals with some form of mental aberration. This situation had to be handled very carefully. Knowing what needs to be done is one thing. Trying to help a Judge when he doesn't want to be helped is a dicey proposition.

The Chief Justice of this division of the court system was called. He had been a law school classmate of Judge Rogers (not to be confused with the "Rogers Orders" for psychotropic medications in Massachusetts) and thought he could reach Quinn. He was also in contact with another friend at Brigham and Women's Hospital in Boston. Together, they approached Quinn, trying to reason with him.

When it became obvious that their attempt was not working, the Doctor from B&W called for restraints and with a Judicial Order in hand, Judge Rogers was sent to McLean Hospital in Belmont... a leading institution in caring for those with brain disorders. So here was a man with Frontal Lobe Dementia. It only got worse!

Frontotemporal Lobe Dementia (FTD) is characterized by early psychiatric symptoms followed later by cognitive impairments. Frontal lobe syndrome is the presenting symptomatology: apathy, poor social judgment and bizarre behavior. Paranoia and suspiciousness may appear. Executive function (the role of the frontal lobe) is badly impaired. The ability to use good judgment and understand sequential actions (taking several steps to conclude an action) is often seriously damaged. There are several types of disorders under this mantle. "Paranoia and Memory Loss/Frontal Lobe Dementia" is the term used by the Department of Neurology and Pharmacology at the Memory Disorders Clinic of the Medical College of Wisconsin. They point out that it is difficult to delineate between various types: Pick's disease is another type, often seen with Alzheimer's.

S T Steve Tomaski—Huntington's Disease

Like Woodie Guthrie, who was best known as a folk singer/chronicler of the conditions during the Great Depression and later known as the poster man for Huntington's chorea or HD, Steve was a musician. Most of his life was spent in the Appalachia mountain areas, once again, like Guthrie. He came north in the 80s to take care of his sister who lived in what we natives call "West County." [That is a group of very small towns, populated by old Yankee families, back-to-nature folk who moved here in the 1960s, and professionals from Boston and New York, who found out that there was a little bit of heaven in western Massachusetts.]

Steve was 50 at the time and thought he had 'missed the genetic bullet' causing HD. His sister had early onset Alzheimer's and her progress through this form of dementia was slower than most. She was capable of caring for herself to some extent.

Problems arose when Steve began to show mood swings, signs of depression and irritability. He forgot to give his sister breakfast and became irate when she complained.

Steve's eldest daughter lived nearby and she called the local hospital to learn what services were available. When she decided to move in with her father and aunt, her eyes were opened to a situation which had been hidden from her. It needed more than services: it needed a major overhaul!

Steve was moved into a nearby Veteran's Administration Medical Center which had a unit for patients with HD; her aunt moved to a long term care facility and died shortly thereafter. Steve still lives at the USVA Medical Center in Leeds.

This case brought to our attention the lack of services in the community for individuals under the age of 65. It appears that most in home services are keyed toward the old-old adults, and primarily in the poverty level. Even in a geographic area where Woodie's son, Arlo, and his family, are very involved in community health projects in the hill towns of west county, as well as their work in raising awareness of Huntington's disease, we learned in our search that caring for a HD patient without a twenty-four hour, seven days a week caregiver, is an impossibility. At one time, I remember a man who had been placed in what was actually a boarding house, existing under the name of an assisted living facility. There was no twenty-four hour "responsible person" in the building. Obviously, there was no nursing care, and no medical director. This situation may be occurring in many parts of the United States. When you have seen a late stage HD patient, often with dementia at this stage, you can understand why so many in the general public are taken aback, perhaps even scared, to see someone in the final stages.

Huntington's results from a genetically programmed degeneration of brain cells in certain parts of the brain. This causes uncontrolled movements, loss of intellectual faculties and emotional disturbance. A familial disease, it is passed from parent to child through a mutation in a normal gene. Each child of an HD parent has a 50

– 50 chance of inheriting the HD gene. Early symptoms include moodswings, depression, irritability, trouble driving, learning new things, making a decision. With progression, the person may have difficulty feeding and swallowing. The genetic test, with complete medical history, helps with diagnosis. There is no cure. Family members should have the test to determine if they carry the gene. As one researcher explained, if people are tested before having children, this disease could be stopped cold in that family line.

U V Una Vasquez—Klüver-Bucy Syndrome

I did NOT make this up!

Una had been placed in a long term care facility outside Boston. Her admitting diagnosis was Alzheimer's disease, variant (ADv). Oh, right! Someone goofed and this form of temporal lobe disorder was not on the screen. The staff soon recognized that Una had something all right, but it didn't look like Alzheimer's.

She put everything in her mouth. Everything. You can substitute your own "thing" in this case. She touched everything, too. She became the "Vamp" of the unit. Males, females, it didn't matter. She went after them. Then someone got the bright idea of sending her to McLeans to see if they had any clue as to what was going on. They did. [You may remember an earlier reference to McLean Hospital in Belmont, Massachusetts.]

Klüver-Bucy (KB) is a neurobehavioral syndrome associated with bilateral medial temporal lobe dysfunction. Symptoms include oral "exploratory" behavior, hypersexuality, memory disorders, loss of normal fear and danger responses, seizures and inability to recognize objects or faces. It may result from cerebral trauma, infections, Alzheimer's, Pick's dementia or cerebrovascular disorders as well as herpes encephalitis.

McLean Hospital, one of the leading psychiatric institutions in New England (or the USA for that matter) has an extensive Geropsychiatric program and can give you information on any type of disorder, no matter how rare.

KB, or a variant thereof, has been seen in numerous residents of long term care facilities, and often is mistaken for an alcoholic dementia. There is no cure. While not life threatening, the patients can be difficult to manage, as you can easily see! Drug therapy is the only treatment available for supportive therapy. Obviously, with a damaged brain, behavioral modification is useless. By modifying the behavior of the caregiver, however, that chore can be less dreadful.

There are a number of disorders considered to be rare. The problem is that too many of these appear to be part of a dementia syndrome and often in patients with Down syndrome or a similar developmental disorder.

There are several seemingly odd behaviors seen in these forms of dementia. It has been known for some time that those with trisomy 21, the genetic cause of Down, will develop Alzheimer's disease by middle age. The course of the disease, too, is much shorter, often causing death during their 50s or early 60s.

While Klüver-Bucy itself may not be diagnosed, there are similar behaviors such as putting everything in the mouth, including small decorator-type soaps which may be mistaken for candy. Wax fruit or plastic decorations used during a holiday period may be chewed upon and sometimes swallowed. Caregivers must always be vigilant when there is an impaired person in the home.

Childproofing the house applies to dementia patients as well as toddlers. We'll talk more on this in a separate chapter called "What Now?"

W Y Walt Yankowski—Lewy Body Dementia

Several years ago, a woman came up to me at the Fall Conference of the Western Mass. Chapter of the Alzheimer's Association. I was president of the Chapter at the time, as well as an Alzheimer's Clinician. Three other women and I started the series of conferences some 14 years previously. The event I mention today was, in my mind, the final chapter in that endeavor. Now that the Massachusetts Chapter is combined, there is no conference in the western part of the State for professionals. The 'really big shue' a-la Ed Sullivan, is now held in May in the eastern past of the State and is known as the *Map Through The Maze*. If any readers would be interested in attending this extravaganza, contact the Alzheimer's Association now located in Watertown. I can guarantee this conference covers all the bases for professionals as well as caregivers and delves into more subjects than I could list here. New Englanders are well aware of the "Map Through The Maze."

My story... anyhow, Mrs. Walt Yankowski was in tears. He husband was in a nursing home and all the doctors told her was that her husband had Lewy Body disease. Admittedly, there wasn't much information available at the time but we told her that Lewy was Alzheimer's first cousin, somewhat like that Binswanger thing. The question usually is: is it Parkinson's or Alzheimers?

Walt was a perfect example. He had a problem with both memory and language; he couldn't carry out simple actions; he seemed to have no ability to reason, AND he couldn't judge distances. He had the shuffling gait, tremor and rigidity of Parkinson's.

A doctor in their community thought to give him some Parkinsonian drugs, hoping that they would help the movement disorder. Big Mistake! Those drugs caused increased symptoms of hallucinations and delusions. On top of those symptoms are all those associated with Alzheimer's. It is NOT a nice disorder

Dementia with Lewy Bodies (DLB) is the second most frequent cause of dementia in elderly adults. That is the listing in several surveys as of midsummer of 2005. I'm sure many such divisions of commonality will list Vascular dementia, or mixed Vascular/Alzheimer, or even the dementia connected to alcohol. I have seen data listing alcohol as being a cause of dementia even in so-called "social drinkers".

DLB is a neurodegenerative disorder associated with abnormal structures (Lewy bodies... similar to the findings of plaque) found in certain areas of the brain. Because these structures, as well as many of the symptoms of DLB are associated with both Parkinson's and Alzheimer's, we do not yet know whether DLB is a distinct entity or a variant of AD and PD.

You will see loss of spontaneous movement, rigidity, tremor, shuffling gait, plus acute confusion, loss of memory and a fluctuation in cognition. Visual hallucinations may be the FIRST symptom noted and patients may also have other psychiatric disturbances like delusions and depression.

Onset usually occurs in older adults, although younger people may have it as well. Certain atypical antipsychotics work fairly well. Others can be a problem. There is no cure.

You can readily see why there has been confusion surrounding this disorder. The more I pick up information from Alzheimer related forums, conferences and printed media, the more I tend to believe that those scientists who listed over 250 causes weren't far from the mark!

While we now know the composition of the 'senile plaques' described by Alois Alzheimer is a protein known as β-amyloid, we haven't yet uncovered the hidden mysteries of the 1912 discovery of Dr. Frederich Lewy. But his 'bodies' are certainly being well studied some 94 years later!

The Alphabet Soup: Reversed
(You will notice that we have started another type of alphabetical order)

B A Betty Android —Lupus: Neurologic Sequelae

Betty was in her early 20s when she had her first "attack" of Lupus. Now known as "systemic lupus erythematosus" or SLE, it is no longer just that thing with the butterfly rash over the face and nose. When we first met her, she was in her early 50s and had experienced various fluctuating symptoms all her life since the first episode.

Betty's husband, Lloyd, told us that Betty had gone through kidney and lung problems, had been depressed now and then, and now was exhibiting psychologic changes that no one seemed to be able to explain.

While their two children were now grown and out on their own, they lived in the area and helped him care for Betty. But Betty had weird symptoms. She couldn't remember how to turn on the TV. Lloyd's cooking was mostly heated TV dinners. Betty had no idea how to run a microwave and as for the computer, which had been a form of contact with the outside world for her, was now more problematic than turning on a lamp. What was going on?

Welcome to the wonderful world of Neurological Sequelae of Lupus. Lupus is a disorder of the immune system in which there is an increased production of abnormal antibodies that attack the body's tissues and organs. It can affect the joints, skin, kidney, lung, heart, nervous system and blood vessels. Lupus can cause neurological disorders such as cognitive dysfunction, organic brain syndrome, peripheral neuropathies, sensory neuropathy, psychological problems including personality changes, paranoia, mania and schizophrenia, seizures, paralysis and stroke.

Not all patients experience all symptoms, but because of damage to arteries, a form similar to vascular dementia can occur as well as symptoms similar to Alzheimer's. Lupus is chronic and relapsing, often with long periods of remission. When Lupus is combined with other health problems such as heart and lung diseases, the outcome is more severe.

Lloyd had been attending a support group in another city and had many friends who were also caregivers. One evening, he took his adult children with him to the meeting, feeling that they should have a clearer picture of their mother's illness.

The word LUPUS has its own psychological connotation. Most people think of the disorder as just that 'thing when you can't go in the sun much… or something like that".

Betty had certainly gone way beyond that stage and her children needed more answers than what they had gleaned while caring for their mother. They needed to know the "how comes" concerning her inability to remember, to follow directions, to interact with people. They wanted to know whether she had Alzheimer's.

Serendipity is the word: "Finding something unexpected and useful while looking for something else entirely" so says Google.

Follow this one; The Boston Channel, the marvelously complete website of Channel 5, WCVB in, of course, The Hub of the Universe (look *that one* up) had news today of "*Study Links Fat In Bloodstream To Heart Problems*".

The fat in question, or under discussion, was 'an oxidized *phospholipid*'according to the primary researcher, Dr. Sotirio Tsimikas at the University of California, San Diego.

The serendipity connection: I was checking out new research on the connection of Lupus and dementia. I came upon a paper published in the journal *Rheumatology* of September 14, 2004. I am listing this site for professionals who might like to read of the connection between dementia and antiphospholipid syndrome.

D C Donald Chapin—Mitochondrial Myopathies

I know… you're ready to throw this book away! Oxidized Phospholipids and now mitochondrialmyopa thieswhatiswrongwiththiswoman ?

Back to reality. Don was in his early 50s when I first heard this story. He was in a long term care facility and his family was very supportive, not unlike families dealing with muscular dystrophic disorders. I don't know if Jerry Lewis knows about this one, but I'll bet he does.

Don's brother was at an Alzheimer Conference and I happened to be seated next to him. It was a learning experience I'll never forget. He told of how his brother had been diagnosed with Kearns-Sayre Syndrome … which was unknown to me.

It's a rare (aren't they all?) neuromuscular disorder with onset usually before age 20. That was the case with Don. This active sportsman suddenly found himself with a serious vision problem and he was diagnosed with a cardiac condition. Built like a fire hydrant, he had been a high school football player. Now he had problems with his droopy eyes, in addition to other worries.

Within the next ten years, Don became blind, lost his hearing, developed an arrhythmia leading to the insertion of a pacemaker and he was becoming mildly demented. He had been cared for at home by his parents and his siblings, when possible, but it became too much for the family. That led to his move into LTC. The family expects his death anytime. They just don't know when.

The mitochondrial myopathies are a group of neuromuscular diseases caused by damaged to the mitochondria … those small energy producing structures we talked about earlier. Known as the "power plants" of all cells, they produce all the energy for nerve and muscle cells and receive severe damage when these myopathies occur.

The Kearns-Sayre syndrome usually takes hold before age 20 because of DNA mutations in the mitochondria. Since ALL body cells are involved, this one is a true WHOLE BODY experience leading to severe eye disorders, ending in blindness… deafness… immobility… heart block…. short stature… inability to coordinate voluntary movements, dementia and total disconnect from life. One can only hope for an early death. No treatment, no cure, no hope. Fortunately, this one is TRULY quite rare.

F E Fred Elgar—Multi-infarct Dementia

When I first heard about Fred, all I could think about was Elgar's "Pomp and Circumstance" and graduations. But Fred's wife told me that the composer was from another family.

Fred was driving his wife crazy. He would sit at the kitchen table, softly crying all day long. She gave him

144

coloring books to keep him busy. She also said that she couldn't understand how he could be perfectly well one day and a "blithering idiot" the next day. This was one stressed out lady!

He had a mild stroke about five years ago, causing him to retire at 63. He had been a very active man and didn't want to stop working. Fred had a history of high cholesterol and high blood pressure but no other health problems. Now, five years later, he had gone through many downward steps, being somewhat confused, then losing his way in the car (on his way to his son's house) and couldn't "be trusted" with the checkbook. She said that her own father had died of a stroke but he never behaved like this!

Multi-infarct Dementia, also known as Vascular Dementia, then Multi-infarct again, has been around for years. It used to be called the second most common cause of dementia, until Lewy came on the scene. MID occurs when small blood clots block small blood vessels in the brain and destroy brain tissue. Risk factors include high blood pressure and advance age. Symptoms of MID include a step-wise development of confusion, problems with recent memory, wandering, loss of bladder or bowel control, emotional problems such as laughing or crying inappropriately, difficulty following instruction, and problems with handling money.

There is a gradual mental decline, usually beginning between 60 – 75 years. MID affects men more often than women. Treatment focuses on prevention of high blood pressure (hypertension) or keeping the pressure under control after the dementia had begun to avoid further loss of brain cells. There are good and bad days, as mentioned by Fred's wife.

Fred became a wanderer, which would have been a major problem except that he lived in a very small town whose main industry was farming. In Fred's case, he only wandered to one place: his parent's home down the street.

While the old homestead was now owned by a family unrelated to the Elgars, the short trip of less than a half mile was too easy for Fred. Fortunately, the present owners knew of his problem and would call his wife when he appeared at their back door.

No matter how she tried, his wife could not convince him that his parents were long dead and someone else was living in that home. Which brings me to perhaps the most important piece of advice I can give anyone dealing with a patient with dementia.

DON'T ARGUE

That may be a bit radical, but I really want you to remember this one! We spoke earlier about the fact that once the cells are destroyed in that part of the brain that controls the encryption of information... the memory center... new information is not going to be in the patient's brain. *It just won't be there!*

So why frustrate yourself, and the impaired person with whom you are connected, by trying to (1) tell them that you just told them that five minutes ago, (2) expect that the note you left for them to read at a later time will be read, (3) leave a meal in the refrigerator to be eaten for lunch, or whenever, and think that your impaired person will remember to eat… or for that matter, realize that he/she is hungry!

"But she is so smart… sometimes I know she's hearing what I say but wants me to think she can't hear me." Or this: "He's had another stroke. We talk to him but he doesn't respond. Sometimes he opens his eyes for a moment and winks."

Think Schiavo. Terry Schiavo. End stage dementia patients, particularly those who have suffered a number of strokes, still have brain stem functioning for a period of time. Winking. smiling and other such occurrences which appear to be under the control of the impaired person are just that: brain stem aberrations. Amen.

H G Harriet Grover—Multiple Sclerosis

Harriet once told me that MS is the "Hide and Seek" disease. She had a problem in her early 20s with double vision and fatigue. Her primary care physician sent her to a neurologist who diagnosed multiple sclerosis, but then told her that when this episode was over, she might never have another! Nothing like keeping yourself on the edge of your seat for the rest of your life.

Now age 52, she has been having periods of language difficulties. What is that word… hmmmmm Oh, yes. Then it was poor vision. Not like before, but more serious. Walking was a problem because she had episodes of tripping and falling, even when there was nothing in the way. She often felt as though her arm had been "slept on the wrong way" as she described the numbness.

Harriet was a feisty lady who had been single all her life and she liked it that way, "Thank you, very much." Fortunately, she lived in an apartment complex with an elevator and many, many close friends, some of whom lived only a floor up or down from her apartment. She's doing well, but does know her memory is failing and fears that dementia is on the doorstep.

Multiple Sclerosis is usually thought of as a chronic disease attacking at a young age. True. There are single attacks, then remission for decades. It attacks areas of the white matter of the central nervous system and patches or plaques form on the myelin lining of the nerve fibers. It is a life-long disease which interrupts the high speed transmission of electrochemical messages between the brain and spinal cord and the rest of the body. Visual disorders are common and balance difficulties, paresthesias, pain or loss of feeling in limbs, may be followed by problems with concentration, attention, memory and judgment. Dementia may be mild or severe. Heat may worsen symptoms. There are now medications which help symptoms but cannot cure the disease.

J I Jake Interman—Normal Pressure Hydrocephalus

Josiah was a true gentleman. His friends knew him better as Jake. Tall, white haired, polite to a fault, he had a regal posture. I always said he should have been the Chief Justice of the Supreme Court. At least that is the way Hollywood might portray him.

His daily jaunt of about five miles around the town was marked by stops at some of his favorite spots; the Elks, if he saw a buddy going in… the newsstand, to see what fishing magazines might be around. One warm summer's day, he returned home and fell on the lawn. Marian, his wife, saw him fall and came running. He was getting up by then. What happened," she asked. He couldn't think of anything. He said that he might have not been looking where he was going. From that day to his death, five years elapsed.

The three main symptoms of his disorder seemed to be a progressive mental impairment, leading to dementia; problems with walking and impaired bladder control. The BIG 3.

Normal Pressure Hydrocephalus is an abnormal increase of cerebrospinal fluid (CSF) in the brain's ventricles, or cavities. It occurs if the normal flow is blocked in some way. This causes ventricles to enlarge, putting pressure on the brain. It may arise from a subarachnoid hemorrhage, head trauma, infection or a tumor (Sounds like a TV hospital script!) It may develop when none of these factors are present.

Symptoms include progressive dementia, walking difficulties, and incontinence. There may be a general slowing of movements or complaints of "My feet are stuck". NPH is often misdiagnosed. If diagnosed early, there can be surgical placement of a shunt in the brain to drain excess CSF into the abdomen where it is absorbed. Early diagnosis and treatment improves the chance of a good recovery.

In Jake's case, Marian refused to have him seen by a specialist because she "didn't want him to have to go through all that." Too bad.

L K Lena Kowalski—Parkinson's Disease

Lena and her sister, Stella, lived together in a small farm town in Western Massachusetts. Pick any one you want; they're all beautiful. Lena was in her late 50s when she started to experience a tremor in her hands. Stella also noticed that her head didn't quite seem to be held in place. Lena was stilted in her walking and all her movements were slowed down. All in all, the sisters knew something was wrong. The problem was, Lena refused to see a doctor!

"There's nothing wrong with me. I'm going to be 60 years old. My mother was dead at 60. So what if I have the shakes. That comes with old age. I do NOT need a doctor to tell me I'm getting old." The conversation ended.

Stella knew of a nurse practitioner who attended the Polish Church in their town and she had been helpful before when Lena got her back up. Stella called her at her workplace and asked it she might stop in to chat some day.

That started the process of getting a diagnosis and learning about what kind of treatments were available. PD is part of a group of conditions known as "movement disorders," and this one is progressive, meaning its symptoms grow worse over time. PD occurs when a group of cells in the brain called the substantia nigra (that produce a chemical called dopamine) start to malfunction and die. With PD, the loss of dopamine making cells mean that there will be: tremor of the hands, arms, legs, jaw and face. There is rigidity or stiffness in both limbs and trunk; bradykinesia, or slowness of movement, and postural instability or impaired balance and coordination.

In about 75% of cases, PD will occur with added Alzheimer's or Lewy Body disease.

In Lena's case, she had mild full body symptoms for about ten years before the dementia appeared. She had been on both Eldepryl and Stalevo, which came on the picture a few years ago.. She went into long term care when Stella broke her hip. Presently, both sisters are in the same facility.

N M Naomi Ming—Pick's Disease

When Naomi was diagnosed with Alzheimer's at age 60, her family wondered if that was really what was wrong with her. After all, she was only 60, and looked about 50. But the doctors didn't seem perturbed when they told her about Naomi's strange behaviors

Her personality had changed and not for the better! No control over inhibitions... hoarding such things as used toilet paper... drinking on and off during the day... and going through candy like there would be a Prohibition on the way. She had speech problems, became sexually aggressive and her long term memory was spotty.

That's right. Her LONG term general memory about the world and current events was gone. The thing that bothered the family most was that Naomi was acting as though there were no controls anywhere; none on sexual behavior, none on drinking, and none on speaking inappropriately in public places. The other attributes seemed to look like Alzheimer's. What was the real cause?

Naomi's daughter was a nurse in a local nursing home. She had heard at a recent conference about Pick's Disease and how it related to Alzheimer's. She heard the words "Frontotemporal lobar degeneration and primary progressive aphasia," in which late stages are similar to late stage AD.

The victim loses social skills along with impairment of intellect, memory and language. The core changes are: loss of memory, lack of spontaneity, difficulty in thinking and disturbances of speech. Other symptoms include gradual emotional dullness, loss of moral judgment and progressive dementia.

There is neither cure nor treatment. It leads to inevitable progressive deterioration in two to ten years. There are medications to treat symptoms but nothing to slow the disorder. You do NOT want to have a Pick's resident in your facility unless you have a large core of workers!

P O Pedro Ortez—Progressive Supranuclear Palsy

Pedro was not a Red Sox ball player. Nor was he a tennis pro. Actually, Pedro was an artist who came into our Happy Valley during the years of the hippie revolution and the "Back to the Land" movement. Reggae was his sound, ganja his smoke and the commune his home.

Happy Valley is a term used to describe certain Towns on either side of the Connecticut River, particularly north of Holyoke and south of the Vermont border. Northampton is the City and NoHo the slang.

His paintings were truly wonderful and he had a juried show at a Northampton gallery. Then came the real world. It was the early 1990s and Pedro was about 52. I met him once and found him to be a gem. Sweet, considerate, quirky, yet a great guy. Shortly after that, my friend in NoHo told me that he was acting very strangely. Even strange for Pedro. He couldn't paint because he couldn't see straight! His mood and behavior changed; he became apathetic, depressed and showed signs of early dementia.

Talking with Kate, my friend, I mentioned that Dudley Moore had died recently. Remember that funny, very short *and very talented* man who played the role of Arthur in the movie? He died of PSP. The media attention surrounding his death publicized this disorder. Perhaps this was Pedro's problem! PSP is another of those 'rare' brain disorders that we seem to hear more about these days. There is no treatment at present, but some victims have been treated with PD drugs to help the slowness, stiffness and balance problems. The speech, vision and swallowing difficulties don't respond to drug treatment. The antidepressants Elavil® and Prozac® have shown to help some in PSP, but NOT as antidepressants. Kind of like Elavil for Fibromyalgia. They may use weighted walking aids (they tend to fall backward) and prism glasses help the vision problem. A gastrostomy tube may be necessary when there are swallowing problems. PSP may be a τ (tau) problem (microtubules inside the brain cells? We spoke of it earlier in describing the workings of the brain) in DNA mutation; this puts PSP into the dementia corner where TAU research is currently progressing.

Just as we thank Michael J. Fox and, posthumously, Christopher Reeve, for their work in bringing about understanding of Parkinsons and Spinal Cord Injuries, we can also thank Dudley Moore, posthumously, for helping solve the problem of Progressive Supranuclear Palsy.

R Q Rebecca Quinlan—Stroke

Once when I was a charge nurse in a nursing home, before nursing homes were all renamed, Rebecca was one of the residents under my care. I came to know the family well and I remember their questions when their wife/mother/sister came to the facility.

Rebecca had been an active woman, seemingly into everything. If she had one fault, it was the chain-smoking sixteen hours out of every day. She had to give up the butts when she started working for a service organization which had a no smoking policy. She followed the rules. Some of the time!

One day, coming back to the office from home visits all day, she had an episode in which she lost her balance in the hallway. She complained of a severe headache, not like any she ever had. A few weeks later, while talking with her boss, she experienced numbness on her right side and face.

Smart boss, she called 911 and got Becca to the hospital STAT. They gave her something called plasminogen... TPA... the clot dissolver. But it was too late to do the trick. That's when we got her.

A stroke, also known as a cardiovascular or a cerebral vascular accident, CVA, occurs when blood flow to the brain stops. The most common stroke is an ischemic stroke, caused by a blood clot that blocks a blood vessel or artery in the brain. A hemorrhagic stroke is caused when a blood vessel in the brain ruptures.

Symptoms of a stroke happening include: Numbness or weakness in the face, arms, or legs (especially on one side of the body); confusion, difficulty speaking or understanding speech; vision disturbances in one or both eyes; dizziness, trouble walking, loss of balance or coordination; severe headache with no known cause.

Risk factors include high blood pressure, heart disease, diabetes, high cholesterol and **SMOKING.** Don't let a stroke be a part of your future. Heed the warnings! Take care of yourself.

T S Ted Sanford—Transient Ischemic Attack (TIA)

Anyone who has worked with the elderly population has heard of TIAs. If we called it a baby stroke, it might be easier to understand.

In Ted's case, he was in the right place at the right time: In his doctor's office. Ted Sanford and Stu Thomas, M.D., had been friends since Prep School. They had roomed together, played the same sports, dated some of the same girls, and went on to colleges only a few hours away from each other. When Ted showed up at Stu's office for his annual physical, he was waiting in the examination room, seated in a chair, thumbing through a magazine on sailing. They both enjoyed the sport. Stu came in, offered his hand to Ted and realized that Ted's grip was almost nonexistent. He also noticed a kind of glazed expression as if in deep thought, somewhere else.

The episode only lasted a few minutes, but that was all that Stu needed. He put in a call to the local hospital, told his staff to cancel the rest of his patients, and off the two went to get Ted checked. End of story: After a time on anticoagulants and antiplatelet agents, a few so-called "lifestyle changes" and stress reduction, Ted and Stu crewed the boat of another friend in a regatta on the Cape the next summer.

A TIA is a transient stroke that lasts only a few minutes during which time the blood flow to the brain is briefly interrupted. Symptoms, which usually come on suddenly, are similar to those of a stroke but do not last as long. Symptoms can include weakness in face, arm or leg, especially on one side of the body; confusion or lack of understanding of speech, trouble seeing in one or both eyes and difficulty with walking or loss of balance and coordination. All stroke-like symptoms signal an emergency and should not be ignored. A prompt evaluation (within 60 minutes) should be done to identify the cause and determine appropriate therapy. Risk factors include carotid artery disease, high blood pressure, diabetes, smoking (again) and heavy use of alcohol. Lifestyle changes can reduce these factors.

V U Venita Usher—Transmissible Spongiform Encephalopathies

When I first learned of Venita, she was visiting from "across the pond" as the Brits say. Her grandson and his family lived in a nearby college town. A sprightly lady of 65, she was a world traveler and she made sure her vaccinations were kept up to date so that she could go anywhere on a day's notice.

After being in the U.S. for a week, she started showing frightening signs. She became unsteady on her feet, seemed depressed, exhibited a degree of paranoia and complained of weird sensations.

Taken directly to Mass. General Hospital (MGH) in Boston, a complete history indicated that she had eaten beef in a small Scottish town about nine months before. The diagnosis, after multiple tests was vCJD (variant Creutzfeldt-Jacob). Mad Cow disease.

After conversing with the MGH doctors, the family knew they could look forward to rapid symptoms including confusion, leading to severe mental impairment and the loss of the ability to move or speak. Fortunately, death usually occurs in a few months to a few years.

There are several odd diseases included in the TSE classification, including CJD and vCJD. The name comes from the appearance of brain holes giving the brain a spongy appearance. The cause: a prion, which you may remember is smaller than a virus and has no DNA. Other diseases include FFI (Fatal Familial Insomnia) and GSS, known as Gerstmann-Straussler-Scheniker Disease.

I think we can all agree that none of us is likely to see the last two disorders. I should certainly HOPE so!

Y W Yancy Waters—Wernicke-Korsakoff Syndrome

A very cool man. He moved into the Pioneer Valley in the mid 1980s after a career in the music business in the Big Apple. Never made the real big time but knew most of the giants of jazz. His son and wife lived in the NoHo area.

Yancy's health wasn't the best. He never really took care of himself and his body showed it. Although in his early 80s when I first saw him, he appeared to be pushing 100! Booze will do that to you. That, and a diet of cigarettes and junk food. He'd tried "The Cure" a number of times, but only came back to return to the same lifestyle.

His son, Ben, tried to be a good son and insist that Dad change his ways. What a laugh! Yancy loved to tell stories about Louis in the 1930s and later, Dave Brubeck... but couldn't tell you where he was now living or the current year. So now he had two illnesses (if you don't count the problem with his heart, lungs, vision and liver) and was finally being cared for... at least up to now.

It's not just the bums in the Battery or those living under the interstate bridges. Wernicke's encephalopathy is a degenerative brain disorder caused by the lack of nutritional elements including thiamine and magnesium which need immediate replacement. While it may result from alcohol abuse, it may come with chemotherapy (prolonged vomiting) and other illnesses.

The symptoms include mental confusion, vision impairment, hypothermia, hypotension and ataxia.

Korsakoff's amnestic syndrome, a memory disorder, comes from a deficiency of thiamine and is associated with alcoholism. The heart and nervous system are involved. Symptoms include amnesia, confabulation, attention disorientation and vision impairment.

In Korsakoff's, patients are impaired in acquiring new information or establishing new memories. Wernicke's encephalopathy represents the "acute" phase of the disorder and the amnestic syndrome represents the "chronic" phase.

Prompt treatment is imperative. Most symptoms can be reversed if detected and treated promptly. Without treatment, these disorders are disabling and life-threatening.

ANOTHER TALE OR TWO FROM THIS STORYTELLER'S BAG

There were good things that happened. I will never forget Geraldine. She was the primary caregiver for her mother, a little old Italian woman who had come to live in her daughter's house. Now Geraldine had four children: two boys, two girls. They were all about two years apart and by the time that Mother Sophia came to live with them, the eldest son #1 was already a senior in college; #2 child, a daughter, was at another college; #3, sibling daughter was finishing high school and #4 child, was at that terrible age: too old to be a kid and too young to be adult.

Geraldine's husband was a professor at one of our many universities. This area of Massachusetts has more colleges per square mile than any other place in the country. Well, maybe not quite, but I can name off ten without taking a breath!

He, too, was a Jerry. He also was away from the homestead a great deal of the time because of classes, committees and as a visiting lecturer around the country. He missed all the fun of having Sophia in the house. Actually, it wasn't a house; it was a small apartment built on to Jerry and Geraldine's place. The builders had made the apartment on a 90° angle so that the main house and the apartment were on an L which had a lovely terrace and garden area on the hypotenuse of the triangle. Got that? [I am delighted to make use of the mathematics class which I was forced to take when I returned to the University to pick up a different degree, at age 64. I knew I would never use the material again, so I had to put it in here.]

Sophia's apartment had one wall of windows overlooking this lovely yard. At the end of her living space was a door into Geraldine's kitchen. Knowing that her mother was incapable of cooking because of her dementia, Gerry and Jerry decided to omit a cooking range/stove when they built the unit. Sophia had her bedroom, a simple bath with tub and shower combined, a small dressing room where she kept her odds and ends that wouldn't fit in the closet, and a large living room which faced the outside through the large window area. It was a delightful place and one which she enjoyed immensely during her early to mid stage dementia.

Since Gerry only had two offspring at home and her mother was fairly easy to care for, life was great. That was until the two aunties came to visit.

Gabriella and Maria were from the old country. Well, actually, Sophia was, too. The three women and two brothers, now deceased, had come to the United States as children. The family worked in Barre, VT, when they first arrived. The father and two sons were stone workers and many Italian immigrants located in that area because the quarries in that section of Vermont were booming. No pun intended.

Garbiella and her younger sister, Maria, were older and younger than Sophia. I guess that made her the middle sister. Never mind about the brothers.

After the death of the senior members of the family, Maria and Garbiella moved to a small farming community in central Massachusetts. Sophia, the first sister to marry, lived some forty miles west of the other girls. Girls? They were in their late 60s or early 70s when I first met the family. Couldn't understand a word they said! I knew a bit of Italian but this rapid fire verbiage in a foreign language with a New England accent was too much for me. What I did get was a lot of picky, picky, picky!

"Geraldine, why are you treating your mother this way? Why do you have her in this part of the house? Isn't she good enough to live in the main house? Why do you keep repeating things to her? Don't you love your mother?" On and on and on.

As much as Gerry tried to explain to "the girls" that their sister had been diagnosed with Alzheimer's disease, they insisted that all she needed was some good vino now and then, some bit of travel, some fun with people. They insisted there was nothing wrong with their sister.

The visit did not go well. In fact, it was all Gerry could do not to kick them out of her house! As it was, they left in a huff because Sophia wouldn't talk to them. And it was all Geraldine's fault for treating her this way.

Turn the calendar ahead about two years. Gerry now has a son in law school, a daughter graduating this spring, another daughter in a college close by, and the young son... battling the ups and downs of high school. Jerry is close to home now, having given up the travels of a lecturer. And Sophia? If there is such a thing as early part/late stage dementia, she was in the midst of it. Her ability to communicate was nearly gone. She spoke a few words. We might call it a "paucity of speech." She had reverted to Italian on and off for the past two years. This is nothing out of the ordinary. Those who had a first language apart from that which they have spoken most of their adult life often revert to that first language in mid to late stage dementia.

In addition, she was incontinent of bladder and bowel, could not walk, used a wheel chair whenever she had to be moved, could not feed herself and had become belligerent at times. It had been a rapid downward decline since the last time the sisters had seen her.

One day, shortly before the sisters arrived for another visit... they didn't seem to care about her condition between visits... Sophia came into the kitchen and said to Geraldine, "Who are you?"

The guilt trip was over. She didn't know her own daughter. It was time to place her mother in LTC. Relief came into Gerry's life. Then came war!

The 'aunties' were coming for a visit. They continued to believe that all the problems surrounding Sophia's care were simply imagination. Geraldine was not taking proper care of their sister. She wasn't even taking her to church anymore. They *knew* all that their sister needed was some conversation and interaction with other people. Those weren't exactly their words but the point got across anyhow.

Gerry had been dealing with this situation for a number of years, as you may well imagine. But she had gained a great deal of strength from her friends in the support group and took their sage words to heart. She would no longer be the door mat for these aggravating, pompous relatives. She felt like a sort of Joan of Arc as she donned her invisible armor and seized her sword, ready to do battle! Believe me, those who reported this story to me were charged up themselves, describing, as Gerry had to them, the Italian Battle of Big Horn. How's that for cobbling metaphors?

Gerry had decided that when the sisters arrived, she would tell them she had just received a telephone call and there was an emergency which needed her immediate attention. "How good that you two are here to stay with your sister. I'll return as soon as possible. 'Bye, now!"

Need I say more? Gabriella and Maria thought there was no problem? AH HA!!! I won't go into the details of their encounter with Alzheimer's. Their continued lack of understanding of their sister's condition was shattered within a few hours.

The clincher of the tale came at the next meeting of the Support Group which Gerry attended. She walked into the meeting… with Lucille Ball's orange-red hair.

They tell me there was actually cheering, clapping and laughing that night when Lucy Ricardo came to the meeting. Sassy, confident, and maybe a bit smug. She had placed her mother the previous day in a special Alzheimer unit in a town nearby.

As for the "Mafiosa" as she called them, they became quite contrite after trying to converse with Sophia, finding that her undergarment (diaper) was leaking, and seeing that she had no idea who they were. Poor Sophia was crying and hitting out at them when Gerry returned. She had only been gone an hour but that hour did what she had not been able to do in ten years.

I wish I knew where Gerry is living now. Although she wasn't a member of any of my groups, I would like to say to her, "Bravo, good and faithful caregiver. You did what you could while your loved one was capable of receiving your care and knew the time was right to make the change which was best for all concerned."

Continuing... and Then There Was Charlie

Perhaps I should have started with Charlie. This is one of the very true stories... true, because I lived through it.

You must first go back in time... to the 1930s, if possible. I'm sure there are some of you who are old enough to remember the Great Depression as it became known.

The "Roaring Twenties" has been documented in every form of media. There were the first of the motion pictures, the jazz that became a part of the fabric of the era, the Great Gatsby novel describing the sociologic and cultural changes of the time. Although radio was still in its infancy and the newspapers of the time were well censored by the publishers, those years which led up to World War II were a coming of age in many ways.

In Charlie's case, the Victorian era never really ended. His full name was Charles Cotesworth Russell, the son of Charles Pinckney Russell, whose own father was (get this) Charles Cotesworth Pinckney Russell.

Our Charlie (Amherst College, 1894) was a direct descendent of the John Russell who came to the valleys of western Massachusetts in the mid 1600s. The family has been around a long time.

The Russell's were important people in business, industry, the church (Protestants, of course) and things were moving along during the early 1930s. Those old enough to follow history and weather phenomenon of that period may remember the enormous flood of 1936 which decimated so much of the New England area as well as parts of New York, Pennsylvania, Ohio and other States. I'm not talking about a spring flood that may cause damage but damage that will be gone by the end of summer. This was one of the largest catastrophes in the area I have described. Think of the tsunami of 2004. Think of Katrina in 2005.

Before all the houses had been repaired, the railroads rebuilt, the roads cleared and rebuilt in some cases, came the hurricane of 1938. This was before such storms had names but the weather bureau to this day counts the storm of 1938 with its tornado-like disaster path as one of the worst. There were no early warning systems then.

Charlie and his younger brother were trying to keep the Russell Manufacturing Co. from going under. Literally. The building was flooded out in 1936 and in 1938. Their company was the last remaining offshoot of the larger company which went on to be the Greenfield Tap and Die, continuing today under another name.

Charlie was a large man. About six feet, two inches, he weighed in at over 200 pounds. He was a great outdoor man, trout fishing, quail hunting … all those manly pastimes of that era. He loved driving his big Packard (that was an automobile) and working, sometimes seven days a week. His wife, May O'Hara, spent her time with a group which founded the Visiting Nurses Association in the area. She also belonged to several other genteel ladies organizations. They had no children. Then came…. me!

Through a roundabout arrangement, I had lived with my great grandfather, a Civil War veteran, who lived with his daughter, Nell. After his death, Nell and I moved to her sister May's place, the Russell home, in the early 1930s. It was like being in a Victorian era once inside the doors. But that had little to do with the Charlie story.

Starting with that enormous flood of 1936, Charlie became withdrawn, somewhat argumentative and abrupt. He was working constantly to save the actual building in which the business was housed. The Great Depression was no time to be trying to expand a business. When the 1938 hurricane once again decimated the plant and, therefore, the business, Charlie became morose. Within a short period of time, he also became nearly mute. While nothing was being discussed in the company of a 4th grader, I knew there was something terribly wrong.

Here is the point of this story: Charlie had most likely suffered a stroke which had affected his brain, particularly in the Broca area where motor speech is found. He could no longer express himself, although grunts and other such attempts were often heard. He also had become very aggressive and finally, assaultive.

Remember, I mentioned that this home was a Victorian… not in architecture but in attitude, mores and philosophy. Perhaps there was a bit of the old Irish at play in addition. Whatever, Charlie was ill, behaving in odd ways, striking out at anyone close by and it was all being kept under cover. We don't talk about such things. "I don't want to hear you asking questions about your Uncle Charlie again!"

But some things were too obvious to close off reality. Like the time that he decided to go for a walk. Outdoors. Naked. Except for his "truss" which was a sort of medieval prosthesis which had a leather belt, a metal brace and a leather pouch (solidly filled with something) which was to hold in a hernia. Honest! I have no idea why they didn't just do surgery then, but, who knows?

Charlie had stormed out the back door of the house, walked through the backyards of the neighbor's homes, following the geologic crest of a small hill leading down toward the main area of the town. Funny thing: I don't remember anyone yelling at me to close my eyes or go to my room. They must have *really* been flustered.

May called Harry, the man who was their chauffer, asking him to please come to the house to go get Charlie. Even I knew that wasn't going to do much. I had already been on the receiving end of Charlie's swinging arms.

She also called my father who was working in a store on the Main Street, and then called the Police. THE POLICE ??? It's a wonder May wasn't thrown out of the Russell family. Victorian, remember. It finally took four strong men to get him and return him to the house.

170

There were also problems with urinating in inappropriate places… like wastebaskets. May had finally arranged to have a tiny bathroom built off their main bedroom. It was no more than 3' x 4' and contained a toilet and a wash basin set into a corner… perhaps no more than 15" wide. I remember it well. Charlie managed to get himself locked in one day. (I think of my daughter who believes that you can fix anything with duct tape and a screw driver. Women know so much more today. Dr. Colleen would have said, "Let me at it! I'll have that door off in a jiffy!") May had to call a handyman for that chore.

Charlie still lives in my home in a way. There is a silver company in our town, at that time known at Rogers, Lunt & Bowlen. Mr. Lunt, Sr. was one of May and Charlie's friends. Mr. Lunt commented at one time that the Russells owned what was probably the largest selection of the Mount Vernon pattern ever seen in one house. I have the silver; I have the reminder of Charlie's anger. Many of the spoons are bent and the knives separated in their handles because of his habit of grasping the utensils in his fist and banging them on the mahogany dining table. The damage was severe. You can imagine the state of mind which provoked such an outbreak of destruction.

I returned home from school one day in 1942 to find Charlie gone. Mumbled, soft explanations were given but I only heard "Brattleboro Retreat" as the answer. He had been placed in that private hospital in Vermont which at that time had bars on the windows and a big wrought iron gate at the entrance. I never saw him again. He died a few months later of "hardening of the arteries".

There were no medications to calm the tortured soul... no treatments or behavioral training... no understanding of what was going on in the brain of the demented. They didn't even know to use the word 'demented' to describe this illness. In Charlie's case, there was a predisposition, according to relatives, to mental illness. The younger brother, Whitman, had spent much of his adult life at the McLean Hospital which I have mentioned previously. The lack of knowledge... and of understanding... was part of the era. Because of Charlie, an aunt, an aunt-in-law, and my stepfather, I understand. I hope those of you who read this will, too.

There's GOT to be a Plan!

Where's the plan?

Every person who is faced with the sudden realization that their loved one has been diagnosed with dementia, be it Alzheimer's or another type, has the same immediate reaction: **WHERE IS THE PLAN?**

I've heard that the panicky feeling is not unlike that felt by new parents as they take their new infant home from the hospital. Some of you who are reading this book will understand the connection.

This is a new experience and no one seems to have a Dr. Spock or Dr. Brazelton book handy. There are, however, a number of wonderful "how to" books for the uninformed. And, believe me, not many are informed!

We don't offer classes in "Dementia Caregiving 101, and isn't that a pity. But, fear not. Between what bits you pick up from this small endeavor and the *real* experts listed at the end of this volume, you can do it. Many are doing it every day in the most compassionate manner imaginable. Some do it even though their own health is impaired. And even though we don't have a neat little plan all filled out for you to follow, there are certain parameters which appear to be common to all cases. We'll try in these few pages to list some adages, some hints and, perhaps, a gem or two.

FIRST This is my own first choice and I believe it makes sense. When you receive a diagnosis of dementia, **start your learning process**. I presume the diagnosis has come after ruling out any other medical causes; I also would hope that neuropsychological testing had been part of that diagnostic process. If we have reached that stage, then start looking for a support group in your area. The amount of information you can pick up in a support group will amaze you! Also, check out some of the books mentioned at the end of this book. There is list of web sites which will be helpful. The National Institute of Health covers nearly every disorder mentioned in this book. While I am a huge fan of the Alzheimer Research Forum, it is quite technical and decidedly leans toward chemistry and genetics far beyond our ken. I know that I look forward with great eagerness to read through the research papers of the week, while realizing that only 1/10th will be appropriate for me. Don't feel yourself to be inadequate. There is also a section for caregivers; look down the left hand column and click on Caregivers.

SECOND   Talk with the family. If you have children living in far away places, get them involved. If they are unable to return to your home, then arrange for a conference telephone call (cells don't *really* do it on this score) so that all are aware of the diagnosis, the current status, and how each member can become a team member. If only one person (wife, husband, son, daughter) is geographically available, then try to have those not at home involved in some way. The days when there were 'unmentionable' illnesses are long gone. There is nothing shameful about dementia, no more than if it were cancer or some other major illness.

THIRD   If you don't have a lawyer, contact the local bar association for listings, ask your neighbors and friends for suggestions, but **get a lawyer**. The sooner, the better in this case. Unless you are Bill Gates, and somehow I

175

don't think he is reading this book, you need good legal and financial advice. Each State has different laws concerning a (1) **Living Will;** (2) **Trusts;** (3) **Health Care Proxy**; (4) **Durable Power of Attorney**, and/or **Durable Power of Attorney for Health Purposes** or "**Springing Power of Attorney**, all of which may be words foreign to your State. And of course, a regular **WILL!**Check it out! If your financial affairs include multiple items in two names or in just the name of the impaired person, you need advice. If you believe that your loved one will be spending his/her last months in a nursing home, get advanced advice.

FOURTH   Learn about medications or other treatment options. Some twenty years ago, I was involved in editing and printing a booklet called "And So We Share"... what we have learned. In this booklet were the names and addresses of local area sources which offered various services. Remember, Alzheimer's had just started to become a word in the vocabulary of the common vernacular. Even those who called it "Old Timer's Disease" had a good idea what it was all about. So our book gave information on Senior Centers, Meals on Wheels, Respite (*now **THERE** is a word which was new at the time at least when describing dementia patients*) and I wish I could say, in 2006, that we have all sorts of resources to fit this bill. Not true. While there are **Adult Day Health Programs,** there may not be one available to you. Some Church groups have attempted to fill this need, as have some Councils on Aging... a part of the Older American Act of the U.S. Congress. It seems as if we just get one rolling and something happens to close it. Many times it is because payment was coming from Medicaid (NOT Medicare) and cuts in National Budgets have curtailed services. You may have to check with the local Chapter of the Alzheimer's Association to get the answer.

As for medications, health care providers today are much more attuned to the few medications designed to delay the symptoms of Alzheimer's. Of course, the 'detail' men/women of the pharmaceutical companies have been pushing their particular brand with great force.

(As an aside, I wonder how many of you in the medical field have noticed that the "detail" person...

the salesperson for these companies… is female more often now? A new angle to get sales? Hmmmmm.)

As of July, 2005, the situation is this: **Cognex®** is no longer used; **Aricept®** has the lead in sales; **Exelon®** is out there somewhere, and Galantamine (known as **Reminyl®)** has changed its name to **Razadyne®.**

A word of explanation about these medications. **They are all** known as **"cholinesterase inhibitors."** That means that when the electric messenger comes down to the synapse (the place between cells where the chemical is waiting to carry the message) we want to make sure there is enough of the chemical **acetylcholine – good stuff** available to carry the electric message to the next cell. There is another chemical called **acetylcholinesterase** which likes to get into that synapse and do away with the good acetylcholine. So, to stymie this take over, the drugs we have just mentioned, known as **"cholinesterase inhibitors"** get in there to do their work. We have the patient taking one of those drugs, say Aricept. That is a cholinesterase inhibitor which acts to STOP the bad cholinesterase from grabbing the good stuff in that chemical river so that the brain cells can continue to communicate. Got it?

Now, we also have a drug called **Namenda®** which works similarly in the synapses. However, Namenda reduces the action of the chemical **glutamate** at receptors in the brain. Pretty much the same action but a different kind of chemical.

In mid-summer of 2005 came news that there may be a drug on the market within (who knows) which will act to shut off the factory in the brain that is making β Amyloid. If you don't have the β Amyloid being made, it can't get on the cells and gum them up! No more 'senile plaques.' This is quite a simplification, but it describes the broad picture. A bit later I'll give you the wrap up on what we have and what we need. As of mid-2006, there's no sign of this new drug.

FIFTH **Set a schedule and stick to it!** People with dementia need to have a schedule to which they can become accustomed. They get up at a certain time, then breakfast, either before or after bathing - and dressing. Teeth brushing and shaving for the men, makeup or hair needs for the women, at the same boring time every single day. I say that as if I really thought it was not a good thing. Well, while it may make life boring for you as caregiver, not so for the patient. The schedule may become your best friend. You can make your own schedule according to what is easiest for you and your loved one. Early onset dementia patients may very well be able to do things around the house, may play golf or belong to a choir. They may have close friends with whom they are comfortable. Your goal is to make caregiving as simple and easy as possible. Your friends and colleagues will let you know when it 'may be time to have Joe stop playing golf.' I have this one question:

Would you let your grandchild drive with the patient?

SIXTH   Dressing problems may come when you least expect them. If your wife has been perfectly capable of getting dressed without assistance, great! Here are a couple of stories about this subject.

Isabel had been active both in work and in community life. She used to play the organ at her church and had her own keyboard at home so that she could practice for the weekly service. While she lived alone in a second floor apartment, she kept it in order and fairly clean. She appeared to be 'hanging in there', as the neighbors said. One neighbor, however, was very concerned about her wellbeing and put a call into a local agency, asking for help.

Connections were made with the correct agency and one of their staff visited Isabel. Her report stated that while she could still play her 'organ' and had a good supply of tuna fish (no cat), her attire was a bit odd. Both her skirt and blouse were obviously dirty and it looked as though her body could use additional care. The plan was to contact a family member and request a consultation.

The only family was a niece who lived in Canada. She arranged to drive down from Montreal and meet with the Senior Care Group at their offices. The niece mentioned that she had noticed her Aunt's lack of personal care when she had last seen her six month previously. When asked whether or not Isabel had a physician or another health care provider, she shook her head, smiled, and said that the last time that subject had been broached, Isabel practically threw her out of the house! The case managers could see a problem on the horizon.

The older woman who has acting as case manager found a physician who had broad experience in dealing with women, particularly those of an older adult age, as she so nicely put it. This female doctor told the niece to bring her to the office at 5:00 p.m. when most of the staff would be gone.

The niece went to her aunt's home at about 4:30, and told her that she had an appointment with a woman doctor. When the screaming stopped, the younger woman told her that there were two others that would be coming to the apartment in a few minutes to help her get ready for the visit.

Final scene: The niece, social worker and case manager sat in the waiting room, having given the basic information to the doctor. They were asked to wait while the doctor did her examination. "Oh, we'll get along just fine. I've had a lot of practice over the years with those who, shall we say, have cognitive problems."

They heard loud conversation and then a thud. The doctor opened the door in a few minutes and asked that those outside join her. It seems Isabel 'cold-cocked' the doctor when she tried to help her remove her stockings. Isabel evidently had a mean right jab! But the real reason the doc wanted help was because she found that the stockings had not been removed from the legs in probably a year! They had adhered to the legs. What might they find by removing under garments?

Finale: She was placed immediately in a respite bed (there's that word again) in a long term care facility for stabilization. There was also a pretty hefty prescription for an antipsychotic drug. Isabel died some six months later of complications from cancer as well as advanced dementia.

And here's a similar saga. Another woman, I'm sorry to say. This one had been living in a single family home with her husband. Both were in their eighties. They had three children, none of whom lived within a thousand miles of the parents. Both individuals had been quiet, subdued, reticent to join in community or civic activities although they lived in an area where five colleges shared the geographic space. There was much for them to do, even at their ages.

One physician's group had a weekly period set aside for the geriatric group. It was an opportunity for those who had no pressing issue to ask the two men and three women who ran the clinic about broad questions. In this case, a man described a situation in which the neighbor's wife was wandering down the street late at night. Her husband was no place to be seen. It was a very quiet rural street and there had never been any trouble.

They were primarily concerned about her physical care. According to the man relating the story, the husband would drive away in the morning and not return until late in the day. They knew he was retired and really didn't care how he was spending his time but *did* wonder about the wife.

A nurse practitioner with the group asked the man to come in to her office to have a more private discussion. He agreed and in the privacy of her office, told her that the man was always screaming at the wife. He knew there had been a large amount of liquor consumed in the house, just looking at the number of bottles each week in the recycling bin! (Just goes to show that nothing is private anymore!) He also said that the woman had several large bruises on her arm and she had taken to wearing dark glasses.

Knowing that what was being told to her might involve spousal and/or elderly abuse, she contacted the authorities who then made a visit to the home. The husband had been drinking heavily as was evidenced by his inability to get the door unlocked, and the staggered steps he took toward a reclining chair. He was incensed that anyone had called the police on him. When the police told him that certain individuals (no names) had been concerned about both him and his wife, he yelled to the woman to come into the room.

His wife appeared terrified. She was twisting her hands, her lower jaw seemed to be quivering and it was obvious that she had been crying. The female police officer took her by the elbow and led her out of the room into the kitchen. Her partner remained in the living room. The distraught woman sat at the kitchen table, moaning and shaking her head from side to side. She was unable to answer questions and it seemed as though she didn't understand what was being said to her. The piece of information which was not noticeable at first sight was that the elderly woman's clothing was filthy and there was a rancid odor emanating from her skin.

The officer asked the poor woman to remain in the kitchen for a few moments while she returned to the living room to speak with her partner. She informed him of the situation. The male officer then asked the husband, "Does your wife take showers or a bath?" "How the hell should I know," was his belligerent reply. "She goes in there and I hear water running and some time later she comes out. Go ask her whether it's bath or shower!"

The female officer then walked into the bathroom and found that there were no towels or wash cloths available, there was no dampness on the shower curtain, and there were even spider webs in the corner of the tub. Her guess was that bathing was not a priority for anyone in the house!

Final scene. It took nearly a month to get the family involved, the woman to a physician, the husband into a rehabilitation program, and the family started on reviewing the legal and financial problems which were in total disarray. The woman had been immediately taken to the hospital where she was admitted for trauma to bones and soft tissue. It was also learned that there was encrusted material around her genitals and a rash in many parts of her torso. While she appeared to be greatly improved after being cared for and had near starvation and dehydration addressed, she still remained severely demented. How much was the result of spousal abuse is still a mystery.

WHAT DID I FORGET?

It's like getting ready for vacation: get out the checklist and see that everything you need is ready to be packed in the car.

Here we go: Enroll your family member in the **Alzheimer's Association's "Safe Return" program.** Then be sure that all doors in and out of your house or apartment have secure locks. There are floor mats which you can place at the entrance that are made to buzz if someone steps on the area. There also is the thought that placing an old fashioned slide bolt at the top of the door may keep your loved one inside. Putting a big red and white **S T O P** sign on the doors may deter someone from attempting to leave.. Make your home dementia friendly. Don't move the furniture around...just get rid of the clutter... wires, rag rugs, including any rugs that may slip... and remember to **KEEP THE LIGHTS BRIGHT**. Make certain that your tub or shower is slip-free. If there are no grab bars, put them in. Turn the water heater down to a safer temperature. If the range in the kitchen has knobs, remove them. Put them in a safe place so that only the adult person in charge knows their location. DO NOT let an impaired person use a microwave unless you are positive that no metal will go inside! Got ant and bug killer under the sink? Get them out and into a locked cupboard somewhere. That includes alcohol, cleaning agents, and other interesting things that might be consumed. As for medications, do as I was once told: get a metal tackle box with a key and place ALL medications, including any over-the-counter items, in the box. Keep the key in a safe place. But do remember where you put it! Inside your billfold/ wallet will work. If someone in your home smokes, (*get them to stop!*) make certain that there are no available lighters or matches which might inadvertently be used to start a fire. YOU may know that we don't start fires in wastepaper baskets, but does HE/SHE?

This would be a good time to finally mention **RESPITE.** That means time off for the caregiver who may not believe such a thing will ever become necessary. Whoa! When you start hiding in the basement or the bathroom to get a few moments alone, you will remember that word. When you suddenly learn that you must undergo major surgery, you'll remember that word. When your sister is being married for the first time (at age 45) and she lives across the country, you'll know what we mean. Respite may only mean three hours to get away for golf every Tuesday … *thank you Kenny H…* or it may mean just getting a hair cut every few weeks. Look to your local Area Agency on Aging (AAA). They will have an' I & R' person who can give you 'information and referral' to any local groups who provide just this kind of respite. As for the larger periods of time, many long term care facilities offer overnight for a few days, a week, a month. There are also times when immediate respite is needed. The primary caregiver has a massive heart attack and dies. The family is at least two hours away. What do you do? Once again, that AAA group will be there for you. It may mean an emergency 'elder at risk' which means that the impaired, demented person needs to be taken care of, or it may mean even a "23-hour" observation admission to the local hospital or nursing home. There are *always* ways to get around such situations. You just need to have those phone numbers ready and placed in a prominent place (like next to the phone?).

Retrogenesis: This subject was mentioned pages ago when I was praising Dr. Barry Reisberg for his Global Deterioration Scale. His later contribution to help caregivers was to tell them that … as a child gains certain abilities from infancy to toddler including standing, walking, speaking, and bodily functions, so too, the patient with dementia will lose those same milestones of growth in reverse order.

The Reisberg GDS is listed in the reference pages and can be downloaded from his website.

Now: I promised an update on Alice and her daughter and Carla, the friend. All went fairly well with the plan in place. Alice was complaining about abdominal pains when the family visited during the summer following the interventions. She seemed quite well-adjusted to her new life and the medications she had been taking, Aricept® and Namenda® had been helpful in maintaining her level of loss.

The grandkids were happy to see the personality of their grandmother was what they had known her to be, albeit a quieter person.

When Eliza was visiting, she took her mother to the doctor. Seeing that testing was in order, Alice spent two days in the hospital. I am sorry to report that her illness was caused by pancreatic cancer. Alice lived only three more weeks. But her time from diagnosis of dementia to her death had been handled with great care, making certain that her life would give her a degree of comfort, supported by those who loved her.

So let's close this rather long missive. My friends tell me that my written messages tend to be exceedingly verbose, but still have a certain flow that keeps the reader looking for more. I hope that has been true.

The most important message I would give you is this: Take care of yourself; have a special friend or relative on whom you can call just to talk or complain. That one person may do more to keep your sanity and relieve your stress than anyone else in the world.

Lastly… this, too, shall pass. If you are a religious – spiritual person, keep that connection. If the old Celtic traditions are more to your liking, let Mother Earth be your companion. The Indigenous Peoples of our Country have strong beliefs in the goodness of all that is around us. Brother Sun and Sister Moon. We cannot be conquered, even by dementia, if we are true to our own core.

Peace to you all.

SOURCES... RESOURCES... ON LINE SITES

Alzheimer's Disease: A Handbook for Caregivers, Third Edition Handy, Turnbull, Edwards and Lancaster Mosby, 1997

One family member liked this book so much, he bought his own copy. A good resource to learn what the technical jargon means. Well done.

Brain Failure: An Introduction to Current Concepts of Senility Barry Reisberg, M.D. Free Press, 1981.

Yes, I know. It's old. But Reisberg is good no matter when he writes. A geriatric psychiatrist and psychopharmacologist, he is Clinical Director of New York University's Aging and Dementia Research Center and is Professor of Psychiatry at NYU School of Medicine. Using Google, you can download his **Global Deterioration Scale.**

Clinical Diagnosis and Management of Alzheimer's Disease Serge Gauthier, MD FRCP (C) McGill Centre for Studies on Aging.Editor. Canadian Group Martin Dunitz, Ltd. 1996

A marvelous tome… and it weighs it! More academic than others, but should you come across a copy, you'll have a grand time just learning!

The Loss of Self Donna Cohen, Ph.D., and Carl Eisdorfer, Ph.D., M.D.Penguin Books, NY 1987

Another old but good. This volume touches on all that is in our hearts as we care for the disabled. This one is truly a family resource.

The 36-Hour Day Nancy L. Mace, J.A., and Peter V. Rabins, M.D., M.P.H.

The Grand Daddy of Alzheimer Care Books. The 36-Hour has been the Gold Standard for Alzheimer caregiving since it first came out in 1981. There may be another revision since '91. I had half a dozen copies in my private library and I'm down to one. It's that good!

Here are a few sites worth looking at _www.alz.org_

Of course we have to start with the office in Chicago. Information on just about anything you want to know from the **Alzheimer's Association**

The Alzheimer Research Forum Foundation: 82 Devonshire St., S2 Boston, MA 02109 _www.alzforum. com_

Medication information: _www.fda.gov/medwatch_

The Harvard Health E-Newsletter _www.Harvardh ealth@atmedicausa.com_ courtesy of MerckSource

The Merck Manual of Geriatrics _www.mercksource. com_

American Geriatrics_www.americangeriatrics.org/ education/forum/dementia/shtml._

Rutgers University (Google and click on) _Memory Loss and the Brain_

HealthyPlace.com _HealthyPlace.com_ **then click on Psychopathology of Frontal Lobe Syndromes**

For Fact Sheets on Prescription medication. Used by older adults: _www.medscape.com_ **(view article as above)**

Enchanted Learning *www.EnchantedLearning.com*
Click on: *Explore the Brain and The Brain Glossary*

"A Link Between Oxidized LDL and Coronary Artery Disease" *New England Journal of Medicine* **Sotirio Tsimikas, M.D. 7/7/05**

The Big Source: For nearly everything *National Institutes for Health* (NIH)

ABOUT THE AUTHOR

The author has worn many hats throughout her lifetime. She's been a singer, trained in music since her sixth birthday, culminating in study under Mm. M. at the Juilliard School. She's been an artist, both in oils and in her own medium, single thread embroidery painting.

The column on Alzheimer's referred to in the book has appeared monthly since 1996 in The Good Life, published by the Franklin County Home Care Corporation.

She worked in advertising in the 1950's after time spent at Manhattanville College and at the Katharine Gibbs School in New York City in the 40s.

Following her marriage and the arrival of five children, she returned to school, receiving a degree in nursing at age 52. Not finished with the educational segments of her life, she received a B.A. in Gerontology and Public Policy from the University of Massachusetts, Amherst in 1993… at age 64.

That year she completed requirements as a registered nurse, certified in gerontology.

Her devotion to the field of dementia, with Alzheimer's as the primary focus, has been a lifelong learning experience. Since the mid-1980s, she had presented workshops, lectures, and some rather off-the-wall talks in all the New England States.

Printed in the United States
72174LV00001B/31-129

9 781425 985813